How to Say Yes When Your Body Says No

Discover the Silver Lining in Life's Toughest Health Challenges

Dr. Lee Jampolsky

HAMPTON ROADS

Cover design by Jim Warner
Cover photograph © Wave Break Media Ltd.
Interior design by Jane Hagaman
Author photograph by Holly Lee

Hampton Roads Publishing Company, Inc.
Charlottesville, VA 22906
Distributed by Red Wheel/Weiser, LLC

ISBN: 978-1-57174-664-1

Printed in the United States of America

For Tomas Vieira, who taught, and continues to teach, that even under the most difficult circumstances, one can love more deeply and be taken to truth.

Contents

Introduction

Saying Yes to Life

This book has one primary purpose: to help you find freedom, health, growth, and spiritual solidity during even the most challenging physical condition by helping you become aware of your inner teacher, our undisturbed core and depth that is always available to us and is the source of true well-being, when we learn to listen to and trust it.

I call coming to that awareness *saying yes to Life.*

What Is Life?

You'll see that I capitalize the word *Life.* I do that very deliberately to distinguish it from *life,* meaning simply existence. *Life,* capitalized, is a power greater than ourselves yet also within ourselves. *The power of Life is the power in which we were created, and that power remains the core of who we are.* This power does not change according to what we have done or not done or due to the current state of our body, though we can create obstacles to experiencing it.

Life is our loving, gentle, and wise inner guide who knows the way to what is most important. Especially during the most challenging health issues, Life knows our deepest desires and the decisions we need to make every step of the way through our health challenge. Life is full of infinite possibility at any given moment. It is made up of energy that is forever moving and that we can tap into, align with, and have work within and around us.

This same power that is both within and greater than ourselves can also be called *Love*. Though when Martin Luther King Jr. said the following words, he was referring to the health of a nation and humanity, they succinctly capture my definition of *Love:* "When I speak of love, I am not speaking of some sentimental and weak response. I am speaking of that force which all of the great religions have seen as the supreme unifying principle of life . . . the key that unlocks the door which leads to ultimate reality. . ."[1]

Dr. Karl Menninger, one of the founders of the world-famous Menninger Clinic, said, "Love cures people—both the ones who give it and the ones who receive it." Responding to our health challenges through Love is another way of saying yes to Life.

Who Can Benefit from Saying Yes?

This book is for people in a variety of physical health situations. You may be currently ill or have recently had a serious accident. You might be healthy and want to stay that way, or you may want to develop the tools that will help you to grow during even minor and common ailments. You may want to prevent or reduce stress-related diseases and conditions or just prepare yourself for the inevitable health challenges that we will likely all face. You may also be a health-care professional or caregiver, or a friend or family member of someone who is ill or challenged physically in some way.

---

1 Martin Luther King Jr., "Beyond Vietnam: A Time to Break Silence," speech delivered at Riverside Church in New York City, April 4, 1967.

To address these many readers, I use the term "health challenges" to include all illnesses (physical or emotional), recovery from accidents, or other disabilities.

What Can Saying Yes to Life Change in Your Life?

In the simplest of terms, saying yes to Life or Love offers us a way to positively and effectively deal with what is happening in our lives now or what may happen down the road.

During all the upheaval that comes with a health challenge, we can easily become obsessed with our bodies, worried about the future, and caught in a downward spiral of confusion, bewilderment, depression, and perplexity. It is easy to forgo our inner wisdom and guidance—even repress it or altogether ignore it—when we are distracted by health challenges and the fear that can surround them, especially if we identify ourselves as being only our bodies. Freedom, which is an aspect of health, remains impossible as long as we perceive our bodies as a complete definition of ourselves. Yet our bodies and their challenges, such as illness and injury, can actually help us discover Life—our inner wisdom, which continues to exist and wait for us to turn within and find it again—and, by extension, discover or recover health. When the mind no longer sees itself as a body, forever in bondage to the physical, the mind can be free. This book shows you how to find that freedom.

Henry David Thoreau said that the degree to which we are true to ourselves is the degree to which we pay attention to inner intelligence. By saying yes to Life, we say yes to this inner intelligence and to making it central to our healing. Saying yes to Life is a means of getting to know ourselves—who we *really* are—during the most challenging of times. The single most important discovery I made on my own journey from illness to health was *Let what you are experiencing teach you. Let who you are heal you.*

Saying yes to Life invites us to address all of who we are, including and especially the power of our thoughts, beliefs, and attitudes. Recent research has suggested that one of the most important things we can ever learn is the connection between our thinking and our health. Good health seems to be most people's highest priority, yet most of us have very little or no education about how our ways of thinking, beliefs, and state of mind affect our health every moment of our existence and even less education about how to direct our mind toward health.

Within this book, *health* doesn't refer to just the state of the body, but also the state of the mind, which affects the body. The results we want to accomplish with our physical health require some level of intention and conscious direction with our mind. The good news is that all of us have the ability to direct our own mind. Like most important skills, learning to direct our mind takes practice and motivation. Our health challenges can provide us with the motivation to learn to command our mind with intention, direction, and awareness, and no matter what is happening with our bodies, this unparalleled achievement will bring us peace of mind, a central component of health. In fact, optimal physical health can be defined as an extension of peace of mind, or the natural state that occurs when we learn how to say yes to Life.

Although health and healing are not defined as the absence of physical symptoms, there is a direct physical benefit from achieving this trustful and peaceful state of mind. Research demonstrates that when individuals are less stressed and have a positive attitude, their physical health improves. In fact, those who suffer the most physical problems, including a reduced ability to recover from illness, have a difficult time moving beyond anger, resentment, and worry.

The old, habitual, seemingly automatic ways our minds function out of fear are what keep us from saying yes to Life. So like someone who has practiced a sport for years with ineffective technique, we have significant unlearning to do as well.

But do not mistake saying yes to Life as merely "positive thinking" or New Age healing. To the contrary, saying yes to Life is based on extensive research in health psychology, a field concerned, in part, with understanding how emotional and cognitive factors contribute to physical health and the prevention of illness. Don't worry; this book is not cold, clinical, and full of research citations. Instead, it offers you very real and concrete examples, ideas, and exercises that you can use right now.

No matter what health challenges you're facing; no matter how much fear or pain you may be experiencing; no matter how little control over your health and happiness you feel you have; no matter how worried you are about family, finances, and future; saying yes to Life will not only help you with what is going on now but may also even give your life new direction. Saying yes to Life will help you with your mental, emotional, and spiritual reaction to what is happening physically. It can take you from fear and confusion to clarity. As hard as it may be to imagine right now, you will even find ways to grow from what is happening.

There is no situation, no matter how catastrophic, from which we cannot learn and grow. I know, because I have negotiated several personal health challenges in my own life. And I have learned how saying yes to Life is the difference between suffering through a health challenge and growing into a better person because of it.

I see each health challenge I have experienced as a class in what is true and fundamentally important about life. Though I am not in any hurry to go through another health challenge and am enjoying life in the fullest, I am grateful for what each of my health challenges has offered me. Looking back, I know I would not be where I am today if not for the lessons I learned from each experience. For example, as I recovered from an illness that brought me close to death, I learned how to truly receive love, and a troubled relationship was healed. When I lost my hearing, I learned a multitude of lessons—from the many ways to "hear" other than with the physical ear to having the courage to follow my passion vocationally.

When I faced my first health challenges, it was certainly not with smiles and gratitude. My initial reaction was a mix of intense emotions, numbness, and even denial. However, because I gradually learned what it meant to say yes to Life, I am not only alive today, but also a happier, stronger, and more compassionate person.

Saying yes to Life takes us from fear and feeling as if life as we know it is over to seeing even the most challenging health situations from a place of clarity and options—even a place of growth and a deeper awareness. Instead of ruining our lives, it is possible that health challenges may actually enhance our days, no matter how many or how few we have. Saying yes to Life during a health challenge sets us on a course of being Life-centered in all situations, and as a result, we begin to see the opportunities for growth and healing in every area of living.

In essence, saying yes to Life during a health challenge takes us from the worst place we have ever been and delivers us to the most meaningful place we can imagine. With this book, I invite you to join me on that journey.

Some of the central ideas presented in this book are a continuation of my earlier works, adapted and expanded here to address health challenges. Certain concepts paraphrase my earlier material, some of which utilize the principles of *A Course in Miracles.* The information and descriptions in the vignettes about people have been altered or combined in order to ensure confidentiality. With the exception of stories about myself, or where a last name is given, all names, identifying information, and other factors have been changed. Any resemblance that you may find between the vignette and somebody that you know is purely coincidental.

PART I

Laying the Foundation

CHAPTER ONE

My Journey

"This can't be happening. There's got to be a mistake."

My mind raced, jumping frantically from one thought to the other, trying to make sense of what was unfolding.

"Pay attention," I said to myself with some force. I tried to stay focused on what the doctor was saying, but the sound of my heart beating in my temples and the sinking feeling in my stomach were winning out. I didn't want to pay attention. I wanted to run and not look back.

Then, suddenly, I wanted to puke.

The doctor left the room for a few minutes, leaving me sitting alone in my hospital gown. The sterile environment of the university hospital exam room filled my every cell, every pore. Aware of little more than my bare butt cheeks against the cold steel of the exam table, I stared blankly at the floor, shaking my head. "Shit," I said.

Ten minutes later, the doctor entered the room again, looking at my chart as though I either did not exist or was somewhere between the pages of his notes.

"More tests will be needed to confirm and to rule out other causes," he said. He spoke as matter-of-factly as a car mechanic discussing a needed tire rotation. But the phrase *other causes* echoed in my mind and landed another blow to my gut. Then I went numb. I'm sure I looked as if I was listening, but I could not remember anything else the doctor said.

I had come into the hospital with what seemed like normal, everyday health problems. Now I was sitting on the edge of the exam table and on the edge of my life as I knew it. My life might be forever different and possibly a lot shorter than I had planned. It simultaneously felt as though this were not happening and as if it would be over in a moment.

I was here. This was happening. And I thought there was not a damn thing I could do about it.

Living Unconsciously

Before my visit to the hospital, I had spent a fair amount of effort to get and keep my life "together." I had done a good job of convincing myself that I was living my life effectively and consciously. I thought of my health challenge as severely and abruptly interrupting my conscious, together life; it certainly wasn't contributing any sort of good. If I could get rid of this seemingly insurmountable problem, I thought, I could get back to my life as I believed it was *supposed to be*.

I did not want to admit that I really wasn't living a conscious life. I didn't realize I had become a bit computerlike, with my programs preset. There was little need for me to have much conscious awareness as long as everything was running more or less smoothly in my life. But when things went "wrong," when I became ill, my circumstances woke me up. Even then, I hit the snooze button the first few times and just focused on getting my life back to "normal."

The truth is, until I became aware of the ways I habitually thought about my life and health, how I automatically responded in preset scenarios, how I unconsciously and instantly reacted to a multitude of situations, I was unable to make any real and meaningful choices about my health. As long as I made health decisions from fear, I was making unconscious and lousy decisions.

It was only with the third or fourth health challenge that I finally got the message. Then I actually started to live more consciously, with more awareness of Life. I realized that I could wake up more permanently, more intentionally, more consciously, and more proactively; make more conscious choices; and move through my health challenge more effectively.

Posttraumatic Growth

As a psychologist, I have always been less interested in the pathology end of my field, which primarily focuses on what goes wrong, and more engaged by the situations where, despite terrible circumstances, individuals are able to heal, grow, learn, give, and become better people. In everyday language, I'm interested in the question, Can an individual be taught how to turn a negative into a positive? This question is the basis of what I believe will be an emerging area of increased study, *posttraumatic growth.*

If you look at any severe health challenge, you can easily find people who have faced it and encountered nothing but setbacks and suffering. However, if you look hard enough, you will also find people who have emerged from the same (or a similar) health challenge wiser, more compassionate, and more appreciative of Life.

How can we choose what kind of experience we will have in the face of a health challenge? This is a very important question to answer, because most of us will, at some point in our lives, be faced with a health challenge.

University of North Carolina psychologists Lawrence G. Calhoun and Richard Tedeschi describe posttraumatic growth as "a positive change that comes about as a result of the struggle with something very difficult. It's not just some automatic outcome of a bad thing." My work is based on this. Specifically, our struggles with tough health challenges can bring about positive change, but this change is not automatic. This book can be your stepping-stone to this positive change.

Researchers have found—and my own health-challenge experience, as well as those of many of my patients, confirms— that those who undergo posttraumatic growth are first confronted with the barrage of details about what happened or is happening. At some point, they experience strong emotion, often including fear and anger. Then they begin a much more intangible and subjective process of finding some higher meaning in what has happened. This book is concerned with the second and third of these stages.

My Personal Search for Answers

In addition to being a psychologist, I know firsthand about illness and its effects on every aspect of life. In my fifty-four or so years, I have had my share of health challenges. As a young man, I lived in body casts month after month in the hospital. In my teens and twenties, I was in the throes of addiction. Early in my career as a psychologist, I went deaf from an autoimmune disease. I had the male midlife scare of prostate surgery, and just a few years ago, I was not far from death due to severe bacterial pneumonia.

At different times, my body has been poked, prodded, cut, and invaded in more ways than you would want to hear, including with surgery, chemotherapy, and high doses of steroidal treatment that affected my mental status. I've had bedsores and aching arms that looked like pincushions because they'd been pierced by innumerable needles. Weight loss, constipation, diarrhea, and vomiting alone in the dark hours of the night are all experiences etched in my memory. Meanwhile, I felt fear, anger, loss, and despair, and I wondered how I would pay the hospital bills and support my family when I wasn't able to work.

As I sought a means of dealing with my own health challenges and the stress and emotions surrounding them, it seemed to me there were two main approaches: traditional medical approaches, which left out the emotional, mental, and spiritual components of dealing with a health challenge, and approaches that largely abandoned science. Few approaches seemed to address the very real, very overwhelming emotional reactions we experience during a health challenge, what we can do with our thoughts to help our physical and emotional condition, or how our challenge can lead us to grow.

Yet hard science from institutions such as Stanford University tells us that our lifestyle, attitudes, behaviors, emotions, and thoughts can not only help us recover from an illness, but also serve as very strong preventative medicine. This research has shown us a simple yet extremely powerful fact: Our psychological and emotional states play central roles in our physical health. Studies have shown, and few medical professionals would dispute, that problems ranging from minor aches and pains to high blood pressure, and even heart disease and cancer, can be caused by a lack of emotional well-being. Further, though many doctors are reluctant to discuss the role of love in health, in private many report believing that there is a deep connection between our health and how much stress and upset we have in our lives, or, put more positively, how much we experience the calming effects of love in our lives.

In my own life and in the lives of the many people with whom I have worked, I have found that the effects of our emotions, attitudes, and thoughts are far-reaching. They affect our general level of energy and our productivity in all areas of life. In the January 24, 2005, issue of *Fortune* magazine, Dr. Norman B. Anderson, CEO of the American Psychological Association (APA), was quoted as saying, "Businesses used to think productivity was only a function of how motivated the employee was. Today research is showing that a person's physical and emotional well-being is often a more accurate measure of how productive he or she is going to be."

The idea that the mind affects the body is becoming mainstream. For example, the APA has a public education campaign "to raise awareness that tending to emotional health and well-being of individuals can not only have a direct and positive impact on physical health, but can have an equally positive impact on organizations as well." When we also add the care of the soul and spirit to this raised awareness, not only our physical health, but also our work and our relationships benefit.

Life-Centered Consciousness versus Fear-Based Consciousness

This book discusses the ways in which universal spiritual principles such as compassion, forgiveness, and love can help us work through the hardest of times. But I purposely do not always apply spiritual terms, and I try to use language that is as neutral as possible. When I do use words such as *love, spirit,* and *inner wisdom,* I am not promoting a singular or closed belief system. On the contrary, all these terms point to the common thread that runs through all spiritual traditions and religions: the belief that there is a power greater than ourselves that can lovingly guide us on our path in life, including during physical and/or emotional challenges.

When we are in line with this power, we are in a state that I refer to as *Life-centered consciousness.* When we are not in this state, we are residing in *fear-based consciousness.* By extension, our thinking is also either fear-based or Life-centered. *Fear-based thinking* and the physiological responses that result from it create or contribute to a host of problems and to a state of *dis-ease.*

What keeps us from saying yes to Life when our body says no is, always, fear. It comes in many forms, disguises, and textures—fear of loss, fear of pain, fear of how our situation will affect our loved ones.

Growing beyond the fear I experienced during my later health challenges took venturing beyond my old thinking and beliefs. Without examining my beliefs about my condition, I continued to stay where I was, mostly afraid and increasingly depressed and angry. My health challenge required me to approach life in a way entirely different from what I was accustomed to and in a way that very few doctors even mention.

The first step was to ask what I was telling myself and believing about my health challenge, and what my thinking and beliefs meant about how I would live each day. My second step was to make room for my emotional reactions without overanalyzing them, which meant I needed to let myself be a mess sometimes.

I wish I could say that I got some profound answers during this time, but most of my thinking contained some form of "This sucks and isn't likely to get better anytime soon—maybe never." I still felt scared. I felt like a victim with no choices. My illness was not what I wanted, that was for sure.

But somewhere along the way came a quieter realization, one that said, "This does not have to mean the end or only a bad situation. I can become a better person from this."

Exercise: Planting the Seed

Saying yes to Life is a means of going from "This is horrible, and I am about to lose so much or suffer endlessly" to "There is something here for me to learn, some wisdom and meaning from this trial." This one shift may not seem like much—and from where you stand now, it might not even seem possible—but I assure you that it is everything, and I am living proof it is possible.

Even if you don't yet believe your health challenge can be an opportunity for growth, you can, right now, plant the seed for this awareness to grow. Ask yourself the following questions, giving yourself time to contemplate and elaborate on each:

1. What are my beliefs about my condition, my body, and what it will mean for my life? Is it possible that my beliefs are not accurate?

2. What are my feelings?

3. Am I willing to be a mess some of the time while I deal with this news?

4. Is it possible for me to become a better person through what lies ahead?

CHAPTER TWO

Empowering Yourself for Healing

Discovering Your Power to Heal

I have spent more time in doctor's offices, clinics, and hospitals than I care to think about. I have gone to the best of the best clinics and seen some of the leading experts in the country. In every case, the one thing I found most irritating was the medical professionals' assumption that I was a passive participant in my healing and overall condition. Nothing pissed me off more than traveling long distances to see experts, waiting forever and a day to meet with them, being told next to nothing about what they thought, and having them react with irritation when I asked for more information. It was a rare experience when a doctor and staff treated me like a coparticipant in my healing and treatment.

Our health-care culture expects patients to be passive participants and views experts as godlike. The experts are seen as having the answers, and the patients do not really need to know much other than what time to show up for treatments. This summation may sound harsh, but it is often the norm, as you may have already experienced. Many people don't question this medical model because it requires very little responsibility on the patients' part. We get diagnosed, get treated, and hope for the best. We take a pill, have a surgery, go to more experts.

Somebody else holds the answers, the power of our healing, and so we don't need to do much work on our own.

But Norman Cousins, author of the well-known book *Anatomy of an Illness*, points to a new direction in health care: "It is reasonable to expect the doctor to recognize that science may not have all the answers to problems of health and healing." Cousins does not suggest you stop seeing doctors, nor do I, for modern medicine and technology are quite remarkable in many ways. But I do suggest that you discover your *own* power to heal by saying yes to Life and thus becoming an active—even primary—participant in your healing and growth.

Though I believe that saying yes to Life can and will help you heal your body, physical healing is not the main concern of this approach. Health, as noted in the introduction, can be defined as an extension of inner peace, and healing is about letting go of fear and returning to the core of who you are—nothing more and nothing less. As Dr. Rachel Naomi Remen says, "Healing may not be so much about getting better [physically], as about letting go of everything that isn't you—all of the expectations, all of the beliefs—and becoming who you are." Thus, your power to heal yourself is really the ability to reach a state of mind in which you can let go of fear and discover Life.

What Does *Taking Responsibility* Really Mean?

When I mention responsibility in connection with a health challenge, I am frequently asked if I think that we create our own illnesses. I don't like this question for a variety of reasons. For one, if I say, "Yes, I do think we are responsible for many of our illnesses," I am often dismissed as New Age or unscientific, despite the quite significant data demonstrating the effects of emotion, stress, diet, spiritual outlook, and lifestyle on certain aspects of our health, and the fact that many of the major diseases that kill us are largely preventable. Additionally, I find this question to be counterproductive to healing, especially in the early period after an accident or diagnosis, as it can lead to guilt, blame, and more emotional upset.

When I lost my hearing, some of my well-meaning friends, and even some people who barely knew me, said things like "Sometimes illnesses are created by us. Have you thought about what you don't want to hear?" Others asked if my hearing loss might be stress related, and still others asked if it might be a result of prior drug use. The honest, gut-level response I wanted to give all these people was "Have you thought about why you would want me to tell you that you're an insensitive moron?"— hardly the "effective response" you might have imagined from a psychologist. Frankly, I felt it was callous of them to even suggest that I did something to create my deafness right when I was facing it for the first time. Early in my health challenge, I needed to learn how to deal with my fear and physical condition, not wonder how I'd caused it.

You see, our egos like to use the term *taking responsibility* to mean taking the blame. The ego is that part of our mind that is constantly defining, analyzing, assigning blame, and creating separation. Its primary function is to keep us from our inner wisdom. It is the part of our mind that believes we are separate from everyone, everything, and Life. Our ego tells us that we are only a body and that full healing is unreachable to us—if it even exists.

Saying yes to Life doesn't begin with us looking for something on which to blame our health challenge, but rather with focusing on what is going on with our thoughts, beliefs, and emotions right now, and what we can do to heal and grow. With this focus on the present, we will indirectly, but effectively, also address the past—what led to our health challenge—and the future in a productive manner.

When I was facing my hearing loss, I didn't need anyone to shove responsibility down my throat. I needed to come to it gently, and then I could effectively do something about it. Interestingly, as time went on and things settled down emotionally for me, the question that arose for me was not "What don't I want to hear?" but rather "What are the many ways I can hear besides with my ears?" This latter question is an example of what I call a better question, because in asking it, I *accepted* what was true in the moment—I was deaf—but I also *empowered* myself. Better questions usually have elements of acceptance and empowerment, and learning to ask better questions is a key part of learning to say yes to Life.

In my case, my better question led to tremendous growth, while other people's ego questions made me feel only blamed and angry. Timing is everything. Saying yes to Life does involve asking increasingly contemplative questions, but not while we're first grappling with the realities of our health challenge.

When we're aiming for true healing, when we seek to say yes to Life, "taking responsibility" doesn't mean taking the blame, but taking a step toward empowerment. I like to think of *responsibility* as meaning "the ability to respond." Being responsible for my condition means being able to respond positively to it.

In the beginning, when I first went deaf, giving myself permission to feel my feelings without overintellectualizing is what allowed me to be able to respond to what was happening in a way that led to growth, whereas too much intellectual thinking tied me up and just made me more afraid and angry.

When you first face your health challenge, don't try to figure it all out. Make room for what you are feeling, without telling yourself—or letting someone else tell you—what you should or shouldn't be feeling. Know that in the early stages it is important to allow yourself to be a bit of an emotional mess. Not allowing for this now will make you less effective in your life and healing later.

The Fifteen Principles of Saying Yes to Life

After learning of a health challenge of any kind, you will likely be barraged with information from doctors and friends, and your own desire to find out more about your situation will also likely compel you to seek out even more.

But while you're taking in all that information, it is important for you to consider what you can do to bring yourself into a peaceful frame of mind and get in touch with your Self, your inner wisdom, with Life, so that you will be able to know what to do with all that information.

Saying yes to Life has fifteen key principles. These principles are based on what has been found to bring health and healing to people struggling with even the most catastrophic of situations. Some draw from Attitudinal Healing, a self-healing method created by my father, Dr. Gerald Jampolsky. He founded the Center for Attitudinal Healing in 1975 in Tiburon, California, and now there are many around the world. He is the recipient of the American Medical Association's highest honor, the Excellence in Medicine Pride in the Profession Award. Attitudinal Healing is presented more fully in my book *Smile for No Good Reason*.

Some of the principles of saying yes to Life may not make immediate sense, or they may even challenge your present thinking. On the other hand, some of the principles may ring true for you, calling to your inner wisdom. At this stage, don't worry about agreeing with or understanding all of them or how to apply them. We will talk about those aspects of the principles later. For now, it's enough just to know that these are the keys to saying yes to Life.

I encourage you to read the principles not just with a critical mind, asking if saying yes to Life can help you, but also with a focus on your gut response. Even if you currently find yourself confused, anxious, and afraid, there is a part of you that is ripe for healing and for growing from what is happening in your life today. Even in the early, emotionally charged stages of my health challenges, there was a part of me, beneath the fear and confusion, that was hungry for wisdom, depth, and truth. Since then, I have seen that this wisdom fell into three areas: physical, mental/emotional, and spiritual. For this reason, the fifteen principles of saying yes to Life are separated in this manner.

The Fifteen Principles of Saying Yes to Life

Physical

1. You may not have chosen what is happening to your body, but you can choose how you respond.

2. Becoming less focused on the past and future is how to overcome fear, physical pain, and all suffering.

3. You can learn to direct yourself to be peaceful inside regardless of what is happening with your body or life situation.

4. You can learn from your health challenge and become a better human being.

5. You can learn to focus on the whole of life rather than the symptoms of your physical condition.

Mental/Emotional

6. Your health challenge is not the source of your upset; your thoughts and beliefs about it are.

7. You are free to choose how you feel and react, and you have the ability to respond in a growth-oriented direction.

8. Your emotions, attitudes, and thoughts affect your health, and you can utilize this knowledge in your healing.

9. Posttraumatic growth is possible no matter how horrific the situation.

10. Health is an extension of inner peace, and healing is letting go of fear.

Spiritual

11. The core of who you are, your true nature, is Love.

12. No matter how sick your body is, extending Love—that power greater than ourselves—as well as compassion and

empathy, to ourselves and others, will reduce your suffering and aid in healing.

13. Forgiveness is essential to health, growth, and healing. Excessive worry about the future and being angry or guilty about the past limit healing and can be overcome.

14. Embracing the present moment brings freedom and is the basis of healing, health, and overcoming suffering.

15. Since Life is everlasting, death need not be viewed as something to fear.

If read all at once, these fifteen principles can seem daunting. I suggest that you not think of the list as something that needs to be remembered or accomplished all at one time. You may find it helpful to take one principle a day and contemplate it often. Consider these fifteen principles as the core of what your inner wisdom has to say, and that these principles are designed to create miracles during your health challenge. This is a bold statement, but I want you to know that miracles can happen and do, often during the most challenging of times, when we need them most. *A miracle has occurred when something that was causing us upset and conflict is transformed into something that deepens our experience of growth, healing, love, and meaning.*

For me, the most significant benefit of finding my inner teacher was going from the most turbulent of times to the most spiritually centered. If you had told me in the early part of my health challenge that the same situation that prompted me to say "This sucks," would someday lead me to say "I am forever grateful," I would not have believed you. But this is what has happened.

Exercise: Absorbing the Principles

Here is what you can do to start walking the path of saying yes to Life: Slowly read the fifteen principles, then close your eyes and imagine that they are becoming more true for you each day. Picture yourself at some time in the future, and rather than seeing yourself suffering, sick, or afraid in some way, see in your eyes a depth and a knowing that was not there before. Ask yourself, What does this future self know? What knowledge is showing in my eyes? What has happened inside of me? What am I grateful for?

CHAPTER THREE

Getting the News
and Going Forward

Receiving the news of our health challenge and dealing with our emotions about that news is our first opportunity to say yes to Life and to consider specific thoughts and fears that can limit our growth and healing. It is also our opportunity to make a choice: Are we going to approach our health challenge in the same way we always have—either by struggling against it or letting ourselves be overwhelmed by it—or are we going to choose to learn and grow within it?

Why We're Underprepared
for Health Challenges

Before I was hit by my wake-up health challenge, I was an athlete always looking for the competitive edge. I knew a lot about how to stay physically healthy, how to excel and push my body beyond its limits, but next to nothing about what to do when I was not healthy, especially mentally and spiritually. My physical health was a given, and I was not prepared in any way for a health challenge of a severe nature.

In our culture, there is not much discussion about how to proceed mindfully after being diagnosed with a health challenge, or how to manage our attitude in the middle of a health challenge. We lack information and preparation about what to do with our emotions and fearful thoughts and how to access our inner wisdom in the midst of what is happening. You likely have more information about what to do with your car or dishwasher when it breaks than how to deal psychologically, spiritually, and emotionally with a health challenge and all its implications.

There is even less discussion about how to deal with death and dying when it is our time. Fear of death and how to face it are not your typical coffee conversation. Yet as psychiatrist Stanislav Grof notes, "Coming to terms with the fear of death is conducive to healing, positive personality transformation, and consciousness evolution."

Unfortunately, most doctors put little to no effort into discussing the fear of death and its implications for healing. As a whole, the medical profession is uncomfortable with death, and most health-care professionals have little to no training in how to mentally approach it. This isn't a criticism of individual doctors and their dedication but more of a comment on our culture. Doctors attend primarily to what they have been trained to attend to: what can or can't be done physically with medical treatment. We may receive excellent medical care, but we are often left to fend for ourselves when it comes to our emotional reactions and fears about what is happening to us and our uncertainty of the future.

Responding to the News

Because, like most people, I was underprepared for a severe health challenge, I initially approached the news of my condition in the same way I approached most things in life—with an "I can handle this" attitude. I attempted to push my more vulnerable feelings and thoughts away. I told myself things like

"I am not going to be negative," "I am going to beat this," and "Being too emotional isn't going to help."

Despite my good intentions, my feelings and fearful thoughts became like food pushed to the back of the fridge and forgotten about—they got my attention on a later date and in a more menacing way. Among other things, I became short-tempered and had little tolerance for my feelings or anyone else's. Even though I kept saying the "right" words—positive words—I was not at all peaceful inside. And though people tried to be understanding, nobody really enjoyed being around me.

So I decided to not stop any of my thoughts and to give my fearful feelings free rein. But when I did that, those thoughts and fears quickly took over my consciousness like a bad computer virus or the plague, leaving little room for anything else.

I thus found myself in a catch-22: Neither of my strategies—repressing or expressing—worked all that well. If I attempted to push away my thoughts and feelings, they festered and influenced me even more. Yet if I didn't do anything and just let my feelings and thoughts roam freely, I was just riding on a locomotive that was heading nowhere good and gaining momentum that was hard to stop.

Earlier I stated the clear need to make room for our emotional reactions without overanalyzing—even allowing ourselves to be a mess. Now I am saying granting free rein to our emotions can lead to being on a locomotive going nowhere. What is the alternative to this apparent contradiction? In answering this question, I found the silver lining in my health challenge. I found that it was possible to *experience what was happening without pushing it away or wallowing in it.* This means that it is possible to experience your feelings without allowing them to overtake your life. It is a bit akin to going on a very realistic ride, or enjoying an absorbing movie or book, in that you trust there is an end, an exit sign above the door in the distance.

When my daughters were young, I used to remind them that just because something is on the Internet does not mean it's necessarily true. Similarly, just because you have a thought in your mind, a belief you've held for many years, or a certain way you've always done something, that thought, belief, or method isn't necessarily true—that is, it doesn't necessarily match the unchanging truth of who you are. This is not an easy realization to come to. But I began to make that leap when I managed to quiet my *inner critic.*

As suggested above, when we learn that we are facing a health challenge, we need to make room for all our feelings and thoughts, but not be run by them. This is a learned skill, and if we wish to grow from what is happening, it is essential that we practice it.

If we watch our mind and emotions, we'll see that what makes us afraid and ineffective is not our physical condition or our emotions themselves, but the commentary that our inner critic (the part of our mind that always tells us what you *should* or *ought* to be doing) adds to the situation, such as "Why is this happening?" "This should not be happening because . . ." "What caused this?" "Who is to blame?" "Who should be held responsible?" "What is going to happen next?" "What does the future hold?" The commentary from our inner critic can be never ending and is rarely helpful, even though it may try to convince us otherwise.

But if we observe our inner critic, we stop giving it energy, and our negative emotions will cease, and our positive emotions will grow. This is because beyond our inner critic, the commentary it creates about our health challenge, and our resulting emotions, most of which are based on fear, is the truth of who we are.

As I began simply observing my inner critic, listening to it as if listening in on a conversation at the next table in a restaurant, I became aware of its commentary. I saw how it was always fueled by fear and made me more fearful. When my mind was filled with its *shoulds* and *oughts,* it was very difficult for me to listen to any true wisdom or find any real peace. But when I became aware of what my inner critic was saying, I was then able to choose not to listen to it and to instead listen to something else that was there, waiting patiently within me—Life, my inner teacher.

Exercise: Quieting the Inner Critic

The purpose of this exercise is to discover deeper truth and wisdom within your health challenge. It is about learning to observe your inner critic without being taken for a ride by its fear.

Whatever you are feeling in reaction to your health challenge—and this includes feeling a mess, numb, or surreal—ask yourself, What is the commentary from my inner critic? What am I telling myself I should or shouldn't feel, or ought or ought not to do? What am I telling myself that is either based on the past or the future?

After some time contemplating these questions, ask yourself, If I look past the commentary of my inner critic, what is there? What does the quieter voice within me tell me?

What you will discover is a calmness that exists beyond all the chatter of the inner critic.

As I mentioned earlier, I was very afraid at the onset of my hearing loss. I experienced many other emotions, too, but most were some form of fear. When I asked myself the above questions, what I realized was that my inner critic was promoting a story of my life to come titled as *This Should Not Be Happening to Lee.* The sequel was *How Will I Survive Being Deaf?* Further, I realized that my inner critic was saying "Lee, the psychologist and self-help author, is a hypocrite and weak if he is not positive," and "You will upset your kids if you show emotion."

When I looked beyond the inner critic, my emotions became much less overwhelming. If you were to throw this book away and only practice this one thing, you would find growth and healing, because you are turning away from fear and your physical condition and toward the core of who you are.

To put this principle into action, practice the following: Taking at least fifteen minutes, three times a day, find a quiet spot and notice what your inner critic is saying about your health challenge and the resulting emotions. What is your inner critic telling you? What fear-based questions is it asking? Write them down, and ask yourself, Does this question increase fear or lead to anything positive or healing?

Then ask yourself what may be beyond the inner critic. Take a few deep breaths, and imagine there is a calmness, a peace, that has been waiting for you. Even if you sense this peace for only a moment or two, know that it is the foundation for your growth and healing. Your situation and emotions won't be so powerful and overwhelming now. Remember, experiencing even one moment of this inner peace will put healing into motion.

The Three Primary Fears and How to Free Yourself from Them

Psychological fears trap us and limit us. All fears reflect three primary fears:

- the fear of physical and emotional suffering and pain
- the fear of loss and unwanted change
- the fear of death and the unknown

Your inner critic milks these fears for all they're worth. My inner critic offered statements that stemmed from each of these, ranging from "I won't be able to handle the pain," to "What if I die?"

As you become aware of the commentary of your inner critic, you will see that most fear, grief, loss, and anger cease to have power when the commentary is not being unconsciously repeated. Further, you will become aware of what the real truths are in place of the three primary fears:

- Most suffering is caused not by the situation, but by resistance to what is happening.
- Regardless of what change is occurring, we can love more deeply than ever.
- Since Life is everlasting, death and the unknown need not be feared.

Each of these truths will be explained in depth later in the book.

Watching Your Mental Diet

In the 2004 documentary film *Super Size Me,* Morgan Spurlock willingly eats only high-fat fast food and limits his exercise for thirty days in order to see the effects. As a result, his health and well-being deteriorate greatly. After watching the movie, nobody would argue with the effects of diet and exercise on health.

When I saw the film, I began to think of all the ways people put the mental equivalent of junk food into their minds, not for just thirty days, but throughout most of their life. I began to wonder what would happen if, for thirty days, a person had only "high-fear" thoughts that led to worry, anger, lack of forgiveness, and stress. What effect would this thinking have on his physical, emotional, and spiritual health? What if the person had these fear thoughts for month after month, year after year?

A large percentage of people live on just such a mental diet, and their intake of high-fear thoughts exponentially increase during illness and other challenging times. *If left to its own devices during a health challenge, your mind will default to fear-based thinking.* It would be nice if human consciousness were not this way and during a challenge would automatically abandon fear-based thinking for only healing thoughts, but in fact, the opposite is the case.

The good news is that it is possible to change our mental diet. For me, making this change was at least part of what saved my life. And many research studies have revealed there is a direct correlation between our thoughts and aspects of our physical health. However, just employing a program of positive thinking never really worked in a lasting way for me (or the patients with whom I worked). I had to learn how to observe my thoughts and emotions, which is quite different from trying to have only positive thoughts and is the beginning of finding meaning. Dr. Martin Seligman, past president of the American Psychological Association and one of the original researchers in positive psychology, notes, "If we just wanted positive emotions, our species would have died out a long time ago. . . . We want meaning in life."

Exercise: Observing Your Thoughts and Feelings

If you were to go to a nutritionist, one of the first things that he or she would likely ask you to do is keep a journal of what you eat. This record is important for a couple of reasons. First, our memories are rarely reliable. Second, the act of observing and journaling is the beginning of positive change and growth.

Begin keeping a journal of your thoughts and emotions, as if you were a bird watcher chronicling the various species you see. A few times a day, sit and watch your thoughts and feelings, as you did in the "Quieting the Inner Critic" exercise (page 27). Name each thought or emotion as it comes and goes. For example, you may write, "I am thinking about my next doctor's appointment, and I am feeling anxious."

Try to not let yourself get involved in each thought or feeling; simply observe it, and write it down. Then watch what thought or feeling comes next. Don't try and catch or chase off any "bird"; just write down a brief description and wait for the next one. Name your thought or emotion, without grabbing hold of it, and wait for the next.

Keeping this journal helps you continue to develop a very important skill, one that will become central to your focus and path to healing: the ability to watch your own thoughts and feelings without being ruled by them in the moment.

This skill, in turn, will begin to show you the impermanence of your thoughts and feelings (and even the impermanence of your body, which we will discuss later). It also provides a foundation for pain management, if you need that in dealing with your health challenge.

Seeing the Crossroads

When a health challenge comes into our world, we are at a crossroads in our life. For me, and the many people with whom I have worked, recognizing this fact is hugely important, as it introduces *choice* to a situation where we feel as if unwanted things are happening to us. Recognizing that we are at a crossroads includes seeing that we may not have decided to be sick, but we certainly have a say in how we are going to deal with the situation and if we are going to grow from experiencing all of it—the good, the bad, and the ugly.

Though profound deafness, sickening treatments for the causal autoimmune disease, and the subsequent effects on all areas of my life were not what I'd ordered off the menu for myself, it was powerful for me to realize that I had a choice about how I was going to live. *I had a choice of whether or not to say yes to Life.* Choice was there in the midst of it all, like a single flower emerging in a field obliterated by fire.

Exercise: Acknowledging Choice

Consider whether or not the following statement is true and applicable for right now, or if you believe something different:

I may not have consciously chosen my physical situation, but I can choose how I respond, what I learn, how I am with other people, and how I live each day.

If this statement is true, what does it mean? If you believe it is false, why is it false, and how does that belief affect your life?

Please don't go on to the next section without really thinking about this statement and whether or not you believe it. Deciding what you believe in this regard is essential to finding freedom from fear, essential in becoming able to say yes to Life.

When you feel you have fully considered these questions, move on to the next section. You may find it helpful to earmark this page and come back to it daily for the next several days.

If you decide that the statement above is, in fact, true, then write it down on a card and refer to it often. You will be surprised how this one action—deciding that the statement is true and then reading it often—can transform your experience.

But What Do We Choose?

When faced with my health challenge, I decided that I did indeed have a choice about how I responded to it: I could approach it without any change in my thinking and without any discipline, *or* I could begin to view my health in an entirely different way.

I saw that with the former option, I was just along for the ride and not much personal growth would result. I looked around and saw that most people stick with their existing thinking, if for no other reason than by default. And that method of approaching a health challenge is what the current medical model supports. The passive-participant, just-along-for-the-ride approach of modern medicine may result in someone physically getting better, or it may not. But in this scenario, the person generally stays at the same level psychologically and spiritually or becomes increasingly afraid and stressed in life. I did not want this for myself, and I am committed to helping others avoid it, too. But I am telling you right up front that positive change and spiritual growth from a health challenge can be the hard road because it requires discipline, conscious choice, and learning and applying new skills. I have found that the payoff is well worth it.

When we choose the latter approach, the road to healing and growth, when we say yes to Life, we became better human beings. I have come to believe we are not given anything that we cannot learn and grow from. Yet this opportunity to learn and grow can be easily overlooked.

For example, soon after I'd lost my hearing, I was angry about what was happening and consumed with all the details. Without thinking much about it, I stopped taking care of myself. My life as I had known it was no longer there. The four things that I had thought were solid and unchanging—my health, my work, my financial security, and my marriage—had all fallen through my fingers. I was so consumed by my fear and loss that I wanted to give up, which, at the time, to me meant not being around anymore. I did not act on any suicidal thoughts, but I certainly entertained them. Had it not been for my children, who were young at the time, I may have checked out. What was absent was any feeling of a spiritual connection or the presence of Life.

One particular day, both of my daughters needed my care, attention, and love. Though I had tried to shield them from what was happening, there was no getting around the fact that they were also dealing with tremendous change. Their parents were no longer living together, and their dad was obviously different, both physically and emotionally. When, because of my deafness, I could not hear their calls from another room or what they said to me, they were too young to fully understand why, and I felt a sadness, even guilt, pierce my heart.

Yet as I looked at them, I knew the choice that I wanted to make. I wanted to be here, and I wanted to be the best father I could possibly be for as long as I would be in their lives. In a moment, I realized, in the deepest of ways, that my illness, my deafness, my life situation, had not affected in any way my ability to love. In fact, *my illness was here to teach me how to love more deeply.*

As sick and scared as I felt at the time, I found that when I was extending love, not only was I more at peace, but also all my problems appeared less daunting. It was not that I never again felt the pain of what I was experiencing, but I had a lifeline—my capacity to love, be compassionate, be kind, and give to others, regardless of my situation.

As I came to know how I could transform my life as I encountered a health challenge, extending love was a consistent part of this transformation. I decided I was not going to be someone who says in desperation at the end of my life "Please, give me one more day so I can act differently with those I love!" Countless people I've worked with have described the silver lining of their health challenge by saying "My illness really made me get my priorities straight, and being able to show and let people know I love them is very important to me now."

I invite you right now, regardless of your situation, level of pain, or worries, to make this statement:

> *I am committed to saying calmly, no matter what my situation, "Thank you for today and the opportunity to love more deeply."*

Once you choose to make this statement, you are declaring that *whatever* is in your life *right now* can help you love more deeply and that the act of loving is a central part to your healing and growth.

Exercise: Extending Love and Kindness

The purpose of this exercise is to reduce fear, suffering, and pain.

The next time you are thinking about what is happening to you, telling yourself stories of what might happen, worrying, and fighting pain, take a minute and stop— just stop. Consider it a short break, just a few moments. Think about someone in your life that you care about, or even a stranger, and extend love to that person. Nothing more than this, but nothing less than very focused and complete giving.

You can also do this exercise at times you may feel very alone. The next time you are at the doctor's office or even in a public place, look around you and extend kindness to whomever your eyes land on. Imagine that extending kindness is your single function, your job of jobs. Or imagine that, in a strange way, aloneness or anxiety triggers in you an autoresponse of kindness.

Extending kindness in this way is an extremely effective tool in reducing suffering as well, such as when you're undergoing medical procedures that worry you or are painful. As an example, some years ago I was in the hospital with a life-threatening pneumonia that was not responding to treatment. Due to a high and prolonged fever, most of the time I could not remember anything and was pretty delirious. But during some tests that were very uncomfortable for me, rather than focusing on the pain, I focused on caring in a deep way for the people in the room, primarily doctors and technicians whom I did not even know. I don't know where the idea of doing this came from. In fact, it was not even an idea; it was almost an involuntary action. This may sound odd, for I did not even know these people, and I had plenty to worry about—if I'd chosen to worry.

This experience brought with it a simple truth: *When we are extending love and kindness (or compassion) in the moment, it is difficult to suffer as we do when we are consumed with our own situation and pain.*

Try this exercise and let your experience speak for itself.

CHAPTER FOUR

Beginning Life-Centered Living

> What matters, therefore, is not the meaning of life
> in general, but rather the specific meaning
> of a person's life at a given moment.
>
> *Viktor Frankl*

During a health challenge, our inclination is to become body-centered, focusing primarily or exclusively on the state and condition of our bodies, and situation-centered, focused on how our health challenge is affecting our lives, why it shouldn't be happening to us, and what we want to be different about the situation.

But we can choose a different focus; we can choose to become Life-centered. As we begin Life-centered living, not only do we open the door to a deeper, more meaningful existence—one that teaches us what health really is—in the long term, but we also begin to reduce our fear and suffering in the present.

Our health challenge can be the beginning of Life-centered living, and Life-centered living can be the beginning of a new way through our health challenge.

Beginning to Listen to Our Inner Wisdom

When we face health challenges, we can fill our heads with endless questions—some medical, some emotional, some existential, some about the future, some about the past. These questions are not bad, and many are very important. But if all we do is ask questions, we are probably, to some degree, resisting what is happening to us. Or we might be trying to figure out things that we may just not be able to figure out in the moment, or wanting the situation to be different than it is. While doing these things is understandable, they can keep us from fully dealing with what is happening in the most effective way. A busy mind buzzing with constant questions is *not* Life-centered. Typically, it is fear-centered, and a fear-centered mind overlooks inner wisdom.

To be Life-centered, you will need, to some degree, to do the opposite of what your fear and anxiety tell you, and that is to pay attention to your inner life. This does not mean abandoning all the details, but it does mean *seeing the value* in paying attention to the subtle, quiet voice of your inner wisdom, which lies beneath and beyond your resistance, anxiety, worry, and fear. This voice does not always speak in words. Sometimes it speaks in dreams, memories, and images or in fleeting thoughts and emotions. Sometimes it speaks to us in chance encounters. Sometimes it speaks within the pauses in our conversations, in changes of subject, in metaphors, or in stories. Regardless of how it speaks to us, insight and answers live in this inner wisdom, folded in mystery, as much as or more than they do in our intellect.

Recently I was walking with a good friend who had just been diagnosed with lymphatic cancer. We were discussing some of the emotions and subsequent questions that come with such a health challenge—what arises when we face our mortality and the possibility of not being here for our children as they grow up. Not many tougher feelings and thoughts come with being human. As we talked, walked, and cried some, we came to a bank of the Carmel River, near my home. We stopped talking about what we had been talking about, and my friend, taken by the beauty of the river and the mountains beyond, told me of a memory he had from when he was twelve years old.

"My family use to have a place on the Klamath River," he began. "I loved swimming there, looking at the mountain and feeling the current run past me." He paused, smiling as he immersed himself in the waters of this memory. "I would dive down, trying to reach the bottom, struggling against the current, doing my very best to reach a rock at the bottom. Sometimes I made it, sometimes I didn't. But it was always fun challenging myself and playing with the current of the river."

At first, my friend thought he was changing the subject when he spoke of himself as a twelve-year-old, and he even apologized for doing so. I told him that not only had he not changed the subject, but also that he had given himself, and me, a profound insight into his health challenge.

We have the tendency to fight the current of our life—to curse it, to try to change the course of it, to panic in it, fear it, and try to avoid it. These are fear-centered responses to our situation. What my friend's inner wisdom was reminding him of was that sometimes it is best to be like a twelve-year-old playing in the current—being challenged by it, enlivened by it, respectful of it, learning from it. The voice of his inner wisdom was telling him it was better to feel the current pushing him to be better and stronger, to grow, to discover himself more deeply than he could without the current. Life-centered living meant playing with the current of his life instead of fighting it.

My friend's story also demonstrates how the voice of our inner wisdom might speak to us through indirect means, and how we need to look into the folds of our lives during a health challenge.

Beginning to Find Purpose and Meaning in Whatever Is Happening

At various times in my life, I have blamed my health situation for my lack of happiness, wealth, and other good things. I fell into the unfortunate and erroneous, albeit common, belief that my peace of mind depended on circumstances, medical advancements or lack thereof, what my medical insurance would or would not cover, the impact of my health challenge on the amount of money I would have, or just plain luck. The earlier we begin to realize our inner peace has nothing to do with outer circumstances, the sooner we will begin healing instead of suffering.

Paradoxically, the first phase of finding purpose and meaning in what is happening is to *be with what is happening* and not even concern ourselves with deeper questions. Being with what is happening means being sad if you are sad, angry if you are angry, tired if you are tired, pessimistic if you are pessimistic. Give yourself permission to be—just be—without a list of *shoulds,* such as "I should be strong" or "I should fight this."

Not surprisingly, "just being" is not all that easy. Most people don't like being sick and don't like all that comes with it. Nor do we like tasks that are less than pleasant or exciting, and we certainly don't like the invasive or regimented treatments we may undertake for our illnesses. Yet if we approach these things with a different attitude from "Let's just get this over with," we can deepen our peace of mind and grease the tracks for Life-centered living.

Beth recently underwent her six-month check for cancer. Because she would need to have follow-up scans for quite some time, she was very nervous and experienced a high level of stress and anxiety regarding the procedure.

I said to her, "As crazy as this may sound, what if you 'reframed' the biannual scan as a ceremony where you give gratitude for the life you have lived since the last exam and the life you will live until the next exam. Have these thoughts the whole time driving there and during the procedure. As you leave, regardless of the outcome of the scan, have a little smile that says you know just how fortunate we each are for every single moment we have."

Many people wait for religion, a new teacher/minister/guru, or a trip to a sacred place to have a spiritual awakening. But the tube of the CT scan or the room where we receive chemotherapy or the place we are at this very moment can become the altar where we discover the core of who we are. As I told Beth, any medical procedure can be a spiritual experience of gratitude and knowing rather than a reminder of illness and fear or just a necessary requirement.

Two days after her next follow-up scan, Beth contacted me and said, "This stuff really works! While the machine hummed around me, I was busy putting the whole experience into the context of a ceremony, of being present. Even the hot rush of the iodine in my veins was a kind of communion or ceremonial climax of sorts."

Like Beth, we can find purpose and meaning in everything we do (even those health-challenge-related tasks we don't find appealing), in all situations that present themselves (including our own or loved ones' health challenges), and in all people who enter our lives (even those we may not like or agree with). Life-centered living, the doorway to healing and growth, includes recognizing that within any situation or change of any kind, we can direct our minds to discover meaning.

Psychiatrist and concentration camp survivor Viktor Frankl tells us, "Our attitude towards what has happened to us in life is the important thing to recognize. Once hopeless, my life is now hope-full, but it did not happen overnight. The last of human freedoms, to choose one's attitude in any given set of circumstances, is to choose one's own way."

To my thinking, the single ingredient that most readily brings peace of mind and posttraumatic growth during our health challenges is finding meaning in those challenges and daily tasks related to them. The alternative is to suffer without meaning—to still have the health challenges, be bored or in pain during their many related tasks, and learn nothing.

Beginning to Reduce Resistance and Therefore Suffering

The bad news about human existence is that pain and some unpleasant situations are unavoidable. The good news is that we can grow and become better people through the process of reducing suffering by becoming more mindful and present. To begin this process, let's look more closely at suffering.

It took me a long time to untangle my beliefs about suffering and illness. I believed in a pretty simple and popular formula: "Illness bad. Healthy good. Pain always causes suffering." I have now come to a very different belief system: "Some pain in life is inevitable. Suffering is optional."

This is a very different idea for most people, because in our culture, the two words *pain* and *suffering* are often linked together without question. Rarely, if ever, is the phrase *pain without suffering* used. In the same way that we expect where there is smoke, there's fire, we expect that where there is pain, there is suffering. Because our mind and the expectations it creates can be very powerful, this preconception is typically realized.

Dr. Charles Tart, professor emeritus of University of California, Davis, pointed out a simple relationship between pain and suffering, based on a distinction formulated by meditation teacher Shinzen Young:

$$S = P \times R$$
Suffering is equal to pain multiplied by your resistance to it.

Suffering, an experience, is equal to pain, the actual situation (such as a physical sensation or symptom), multiplied by our resistance to what is happening in the now; our resistance is a result of our mind being attached to having things a certain way rather than the way they actually are. With this formula, we can see that the amount we suffer is directly linked to the attitudes and thoughts we hold in our mind.

When I lost my hearing to an autoimmune disease, I initially suffered a great deal of fear but never questioned the suffering, thinking it was a very natural, if unavoidable, response. But as I thought about my situation, I realized that my automatic-suffering response could change even if the situation did not.

Using the equation *suffering = pain x resistance,* if I had a lot of actual physical change/loss/pain (say my deafness ranked as an 8, on a 10-point scale) and a lot of resistance to what was actually happening in the moment, with thoughts such as "This should not be happening to me," and "The future is going to be awful now" (say 6 on a 10-point scale), I would get 48 (8 x 6) units of suffering. In contrast, if I chose to lessen my resistance to what *is* by changing my thoughts and attitude, dropping my resistance to, say, a 1, then the most units of suffering I would get is 8 (8 x 1).

The doorway to healing and health begins to swing open as you look at your own numbers. Take some time to answer the following:

- On a scale of 1 to 10, where is your pain (emotional and/or physical)?

- On a scale of 1 to 10, where is your resistance?

- What thoughts increase resistance?

- What is an alternate view and thought system that decreases resistance and therefore suffering?

All the exercises in this book help us reduce fear and suffering by reducing resistance, and they reduce our resistance by helping us

1. accept what is,

2. find lessons in what is, and

3. cultivate mindfulness.

These three skills are extremely important and directly contrast what the untrained and unfocused mind usually wants to do: fan the flames of resistance by being very fearful and staying attached to having something happen other than what actually is happening. For example, it is not unusual for a person to have 2 units of pain (perhaps a bad cold) combined with 10 units of resistance (with thoughts such as "Why me? Why now? I always get sick at the worst possible time!") and to end up with a very inflated 20 units of suffering over a simple illness.

Jon Kabat-Zinn of the University of Massachusetts Medical School defines mindfulness as a "means of paying attention in a particular way: on purpose, in the present moment, and non-judgmentally." Purposefulness is also a very important part of saying yes to Life. Having the purpose of staying with our experience during our health challenge, be it a particular emotion or a medical procedure, means that we are actively involving ourselves in our experience, shaping the mind rather than being passively taken along for a ride.

During my own health challenges, I have found that with mindfulness I can handle pain and fear without nearly as much suffering as I once thought was normal. But I have also noticed that when I am not paying at least some mindful attention to my thoughts, I can easily make trivial pains into great sufferings, and fear can ignite like dry grass on a windy day. The fearful part of our mind is always on the lookout for an opportunity to turn pain into suffering. Perhaps the most common way our mind does this is by projecting our fears into the future, with thoughts such as "Will this ever end?"

As you face your current health challenge, you will need to become aware of this aspect of your mind with great diligence. Do not expect yourself to be all that successful at mindfulness at first, because at the beginning of a health challenge, your level of fear, pain, and anxiety is very high, and perhaps the level of physical and/or emotional pain is more than you feel you can manage. But there is a part of your mind that can deal with this fear and anxiety from a Life-centered place, to watch your mind without being taken by it. Do not resist your mind, but also do not be controlled by it. I am not saying don't be fearful or pretend you don't have pain. I am saying don't let yourself be blindly taken for a ride by your fear or controlled by your pain.

Exercise: Watching Your Mind

I suggest setting aside times during the day when you will continue to train your mind to deal with what is happening. Imagine that there is a part of your mind that can observe and watch your thoughts in the moment but not be taken in by them. This part of your mind also does not project fear into the future, with "what if" thoughts, such as "What if the pain doesn't stop or even gets worse?" or "What if there's no cure?" A few times during your day, simply observe your thinking and your reactions. Nothing more than this.

Over time, you will find yourself looking forward to these moments because they yield a calmness during even the most turbulent times. Posttraumatic growth comes from this approach, whereas posttraumatic stress comes from continued high levels of stress and anxiety and projecting a bad experience into the future.

Beginning to Change Focus

You may not have consciously chosen what is happening to your body, but you can consciously choose your reactions. However, choosing and changing your reactions are not necessarily easy.

Our minds, having spent years of doing pretty much whatever they want to do, are initially not very cooperative to any conscious direction. Most of us have minds that are not dissimilar to adolescents; our minds act as if they don't want direction, but they are really looking for it.

Much of what saying yes to Life involves is consistent with the teachings of contemporary cognitive psychology but also includes the humanistic-existential components of meaning, purpose, and love. Suffering is seen as a result of *ceasing to remain in the present moment with whatever is happening* to us. Instead of staying present in the moment, we make up a reality in our minds and project that reality into our future. This projected reality always includes some fear, obsession, and worry, and lack of peace of mind is the result.

For example, when I was attached to my desire to be rid of my deafness, that attachment dominated how I responded to the situation. I believed I had to find a medical cure for my deafness in order to be happy, and this search absorbed most all my attention and energy. Though I was doing a lot of research and visiting the very best doctors in the country, I was not at peace and was pretty much in a constant state of worry. When I allowed this fear-based consciousness to grow, the result was an increase in unhappiness and a buildup of resentment, fear, and anxiety. Paradoxically, this negative shift in my emotions worsened my hearing and increased other symptoms of my illness. In short, my complete obsession with getting better actually made me worse.

Suffering involves your fearful mind, your attitudes, your thoughts, and how you respond to the pain of a given situation. Painful situations in life are not something any person has ever been able to entirely control, avoid, or get rid of, despite all our efforts to do so—efforts ranging from drugs, obsessive control, modern medicine, isolation, and material possessions. The doorway to healing and growth begins with *how you respond* to something, not with keeping the something from happening. You *can* shape and have control over your response by becoming more mindful, and this determines your experience. The goal of Life-centered living is *not* to control all our health challenges, symptoms, and difficult situations; rather, *the initial goal is to reduce suffering and increase peace of mind by mindfully looking at our responses to whatever is happening in our lives.*

Please don't think of successful healing as the removal of physical symptoms. If you do, you will miss the goal of true healing: the experience of peace of mind. The more your sole aim is to get rid of your physical symptoms, and the more you are attached to reaching that goal, the less likely it is that you will achieve it. Like happiness, health cannot be bought, chased, or forced. It comes from recognizing who you are at your core. And recognizing who you are is a by-product of focusing less, not more, on your symptoms, while simultaneously reaching out to a greater good or dedicating yourself to a person other than yourself.

Groups of children with catastrophic illnesses at the Centers of Attitudinal Healing clearly demonstrate the effectiveness of this key aspect of Life-centered living. When young people are actively helping others, their own suffering often disappears!

When we are actively giving, we cannot be actively suffering.

I have witnessed this miracle in countless other groups as well—from adult cancer-support groups to twelve-step groups. Simply put, when we focus less on our own symptoms and condition and surrender to the act of selflessly giving to another being, our suffering is greatly reduced and replaced by a sense of peace of mind.

In my book *Smile for No Good Reason*, I noted that happiness can only happen when we stop chasing it or even caring about it so much and instead trust that it is there, within, for us to discover. The same holds for health and healing—we must allow health and healing to happen by not overfocusing on them and not caring about them so much and instead trusting that healing and health are within us.

All this may sound contrary to what you may think you want, what you have been told, or what you have read. And to be clear, *I am certainly not advocating stopping attending to prescribed or available medical treatments.* What I am talking about is where you direct you mind and what your goals are. From my own experience, I know that my healing happened precisely because, through trusting my inner wisdom, *I had ceased to make it all I thought about.*

Did my physical symptoms improve? After I'd lost my hearing, for example, was my hearing restored as a result of my healing? The answer is no. I write this to you as a deaf man, but I am a deaf man who has peace of mind and is giving to you, the reader, in this moment, fully. I consider this state to be one of health and continual healing, and I am grateful for it.

There are many spiritual leaders—ranging from the Buddha and Christ to modern-day figures—who have demonstrated choosing to have a Life-centered focus during extreme hardship. Regardless of whether or not you consider yourself a spiritual or religious person, and regardless of whether you believe in any of these figures or not, their stories can inspire you.

For example, in the hours Jesus was hanging on the cross, nails piercing his body and thorns digging into his scalp, he was able to ask God to be merciful to those who had put him there. In order to say "Father, forgive them for they know not what they do," his resistance to his pain must have been very low. He was not internally fighting what was happening, because his peace of mind lay *not* in getting off the cross but in extending compassion and understanding in the moment, *even in dire circumstances*. He must have been experiencing tremendous physical pain, yet he did not allow this pain to take control of his mind and Spirit. The personal lesson I take away from his story is this: Despite the physical or emotional pain we may be feeling, we can choose to direct our mind in a way that limits our suffering. *We can choose to love regardless of the state of our body.*

Learning to change our focus while we're in the throes of a health challenge is not always a straightforward or easy task. If over weeks, months, or years, you have found yourself unhappy, frustrated, or angry, you may begin to believe that health and spiritual fulfillment are nowhere to be found and that increased suffering is inevitable. These thoughts can be very self-defeating, draining you of the vitality you need to recover and learn from your life and health as they are today. But don't worry. This is what I was thinking just before I began to change my focus during my health challenge, and these are the same thoughts, emotions, and beliefs from which you can advance in your journey.

All that is necessary right now is the slightest thought that maybe, just maybe, any health challenge, now or in the future, has a purpose: to bring you closer to Spirit and to those you love, to raise your consciousness, and to redirect your life. Just the tiniest spark of belief at this point is more than sufficient.

Beginning to Find Love and Purpose

Several years ago, I worked with a fifty-six-year-old man, Chris, who was in the last stages of his life. Chris had lived a life where he was not always honest, and he had a long history of failed business endeavors and personal relationships. He was not proud of himself or the life he had lived, and he was struggling with dying. He was in a great deal of physical and emotional pain, and though he had available to him extensive pain medication, for some reason, he had stopped taking it all.

One Sunday afternoon, three days before he passed, I visited him. The number of times he was awake and clear was decreasing. I sat by his bedside while he was in a semiconscious state, wondering what he might be experiencing. When he opened his eyes, surprisingly, he looked as though he were not in any pain at all.

"For the first time, I just realized the truth about my life," he said. "The truth is, I am loved."

Where did this realization come from? Certainly not from his view of himself. To the contrary, it came from a miraculous moment in which he was able to transcend his view of himself.

A health challenge can strip us of our view of what I call the *small self*, the view of ourselves based on our past, regardless of whether that view is positive or negative. Getting beyond the view of our small self, or our ego, is important, because that is where Love abides—in the humility beyond the small self. This is also a good definition of forgiveness: the state of mind that results when we see beyond our, or another person's, small self and recognize Love.

Finding that place of Love within is the highest and most precious goal for which we can reach. What Chris realized in his last hours was that *his salvation, his healing, was through Love, because Love is who and what he is.*

Chris reminded me that even when we believe we have not led the most moral of lives, *we can discover who we are at any given time. And when we do, forgiveness happens.* Chris showed me how a person who has very little left in this world can still discover a state of bliss. Even if this bliss is experienced only for an instant, that instant is enough.

After Chris told me that he knew he was loved, I asked him which of his past actions caused him the most emotional pain. He told me that he had not spoken with his daughter in over a decade and did not even know where she lived anymore. I suggested that though he had been feeling guilty about losing track of his daughter for all these years, there was something different he could do right now. One way for him to bring his life to a close in a positive way would be to focus all his attention on extending love to his daughter rather than anger toward himself.

Chris had entered his illness believing he was severed from Love, from people he cared about, and he was wracked with guilt. But at the end of his illness, as he lay in a hospital bed, when he no longer had the time to find his daughter or do "the right thing," he was able to hold his daughter in complete love and caring. He was able to live honorably and find authentic success by dealing with his sufferings in a way that took him beyond himself. He left this life with a purpose.

As Chris's story illustrates, health challenges bring us opportunities to release layers of who we *think* we are so that we can find who we *really* are. Releasing these small-self layers is part of Life-centered living, part of the path to finding peace of mind through forgiveness when we are faced with pain or difficulty.

I invite you to commit to Life-centered living by deciding to focus your energy on developing your ability to become a loving, compassionate, and forgiving human being and on finding newfound purpose in your life, regardless of what stage of it you find yourself in.

Beginning to Trust

As you take on a new purpose—to love more deeply and listen to your inner wisdom—the benefits will transfer to other areas of your life as well. For example, you will be able to release old, outdated life strategies that may have been impeding your personal and career success for years. Releasing these old strategies, in turn, enables you to develop a sense of trust in your life as it unfolds. After life-threatening health challenges, many people report that they feel less of a need to try to control outcomes in their day-to-day lives, and that without this need for control, they feel more freedom and peace of mind.

Through Life-centered living during a health challenge, you come to know that *you* are trustworthy, that *Life* is trustworthy, and that trusting yourself and Life is the foundation for decreased stress and increased health. Along with this trust comes an increasing recognition that we are each fully capable of great compassion and of being a loving human being.

When, in his last days, Chris recognized his own compassion and ability to love and be loved, his health challenge became his spiritual awakening. Simply put, having a spiritual awakening means seeing that your past is not who you are, recognizing that your body is not a limit, and experiencing the Love that is always available to us.

A fearful mind creates a lack of trust in ourselves and Life, which then limits healing. To maximize healing, we need to recognize where we lack trust and why. If we have difficulty trusting Life, more than likely our view of the nature of trust is almost exclusively derived from painful past experiences.

Unfortunately, many of us learned about the world and what health is from parents who were themselves untrusting and unhealthy or from role models who rarely reached us and often left us confused. From an early age, we hear many "don't trust" messages, but very few "trust" messages. As a result, when it comes to health challenges, we seldom trust that there is something we can learn from them. We rarely hear "Trust that you will discover more of who you really are."

A common misconception is that trust is something we can feel only when "good" things happen. This way of thinking says "If only I could go through life with no pain, then I could trust," or "How can I possibly trust after this terrible thing has happened to me?" or "My physical condition is very unstable, and I never know what is going to happen next. Therefore, it is impossible to consistently trust how my life unfolds."

Life-centered living offers an alternative definition of trust: *Trust is the state of mind defined by the absence of fear.* Because trust in Love reduces fear, trust in Love contributes to physical, emotional, and spiritual health. Fear is the foundation of disease, but Life and Love are the foundation of health. A health challenge is our opportunity to learn to trust that the awareness of Love, the awareness of Life, will come.

Beginning to Think beyond Fear

One key shift that can move us away from being a passive participant in or victim of our health challenges is becoming aware of and catching our fear-based automatic responses. Fear-based thinking always sees situations as either/or, as black or white. When we realize we are engaging in such thinking, we can pause and realize there are other options, other ways of seeing the situation.

When you find yourself engaging in either/or thinking, ask yourself, What else is possible? What thinking can bring me peace of mind?

As an exercise in Life-centered living, you might want to try saying to yourself, out loud or in writing,

> *There is more than either/or thinking, and there is a purpose to my health challenge. It is to better know myself now and in the future and to discover Life. I shall focus my attention on the energy of Love that is within me, and become a more compassionate, forgiving human being.*

To say this and mean it is to change your entire experience and life. To say this and mean it is to recognize that a fearful mind and the negative emotions it creates contribute to illness and reduce the ability to recover fully. *Any approach to healing that fails to reduce fear, anger, guilt, hostility, and stress is never going to lead to full health.*

Fortunately, even when we do not consciously choose to awaken from our fearful state of mind, Life, our inner wisdom, still compels us to do so, and it often supplies the means. Chris is a good example of someone whom Life compelled to awaken.

We can, however, choose to help open the door to the wisdom of Life. Each day, choose to set your mind in a direction that will reclaim your capacity for a deeply satisfying existence by reminding yourself there is another way to go through life besides being led by fear and either/or thinking.

Beginning to Cultivate a Healthy Mind

Every thought or action either develops health or inhibits it. There are no neutral thoughts. Our attempts to be healthier are destined for failure unless we are willing to wake up from the unconsciousness of the fearful mind and begin deepening our commitment to redirecting our mind toward Love.

In contrast to the "diagnostic protocol" of Western medicine, a checklist or decision tree that typically lists negative symptoms of a dis-ease state, the following list gives positive symptoms of a healthy mind. This list was mostly created by my friend and colleague Don Goewey, an author synthesizing research in neuroscience.

A healthy mind

- ❖ gives us a calm, clear sense of our own power without the need to overpower others or have their approval.

- ❖ is unafraid, unhurried, and kind.

- ❖ has a curious vitality that is fully present.

- ❖ is willing to engage life exactly as it is.

- is not interested in judging ourselves, others, or events.

- feels no need to change anyone.

- has compassionate understanding that is not codependent.

- is willing to forgive.

- has ceased to worry.

- feels a connection with others and with Life itself.

- experiences a sense of the sacred.

In today's world of constant stimulation and stress, it is not easy to develop this healthy mind. When you add the stress of a health challenge, developing a healthy mind becomes an even more difficult task. But it is still entirely possible. In fact, facing a health challenge can actually speed up the development of a healthy mind.

Exercise: Developing a Healthy Mind during a Health Challenge

The purpose of this exercise is to direct your mind toward peace and healing.

Sit for five minutes with your eyes closed, focusing on your breath. Breathe in and breathe out, with long, deep belly breaths. Consciously place a gentle smile on your face as you breathe, even if you do not feel you have anything to be happy about.

Then, open your eyes, keeping the smile, and slowly read the list below three times. Don't worry if you don't fully believe the following statements. They are equally statements of truth and statements of where you wish to direct your mind.

I have a calm, clear sense of my own power without the need to overpower others or have their approval.

I am unafraid. I am unhurried. I am kind.

I have a curious vitality that is fully present.

I am willing to engage life exactly as it is.

I have no interest in judging myself, others, or events.

I have no need to change anyone.

I have a compassionate understanding that is not codependent.

I am willing to forgive.

I trust. I release all worry.

I feel connected with others and with Life itself.

I have a sense of what is sacred.

You may want to do this exercise several times a day.

CHAPTER FIVE

Initial Decisions

Decide to Be a Learner Instead of a Victim

We can approach our health challenges in two very different ways: as a victim or as a learner. Which we choose determines whether we increase fear or increase healing.

When we first face a health challenge, it is common to see the situation through the same lens through which we see the rest of our life. We often see events as happening randomly, and at best, we can be a passive and fearful participant in them. This view is the victim approach.

The alternative, and much more positive, approach begins when we decide (and it must be a conscious decision) to learn and grow from our health challenge and to be active in our healing. This is the learner approach. From the standpoint of Life-centered living, the victim approach obscures healing, and the learner approach increases healing.

The victim approach is fueled by fear, and the learner approach is fueled by trust. According to the victim, we are like the ball in a pinball game, being sent in all directions by outside forces. To the learner, life is a series of endless opportunities to learn and grow, to become better, more loving human beings. The victim always judges and labels a situation as good or bad and then determines that this situation should or should not be happening. The learner sees all situations as opportunities to deepen our ability to know who we are, to experience our potential, and to give and receive love.

If we leave our minds to their own devices and don't consciously decide to learn, chances are we will fall into the victim approach, if for no other reason than being a victim is usually our default mode when our fear factor is high, as it is during a health challenge.

How I Became a Learner

I decided to become a learner rather than a victim during my own health challenge after exploring the differences between people who go through similar health challenges but have very different experiences and outcomes.

I found that people who experienced posttraumatic growth took the learner approach to their challenge. They actually did not see themselves as victims, no matter their circumstances. This did not mean that they were happy about the challenges they faced, but it does mean that, somewhere along the line, they chose to see their challenges as a part of life that can lift them spiritually and deepen them emotionally. Further, many of these people developed a mind-set that they could learn from whatever happens in their life. This unique outlook often included a sense of peace that others never know. This outlook and this sense of peace were something I wanted for myself, so I set out to learn more about the learner approach.

What I first discovered was that both the victim and learner approaches are learned behaviors based on how we see life working, specifically whether we see circumstances or attitudes and thoughts as the primary cause of what we experience. This was good news to me because, as a psychologist and educator, I knew that with conscious mindfulness and motivation, we can make significant changes, even in the face of challenges. So I set out to develop a learner approach to my own health challenges, even while I was still very entrenched in the victim approach.

It was personally very challenging for me to give up being a victim. In addition to being sick, I also was ill from the treatment itself. I had two young kids to take care of and was separated from my wife. I had no job because of my illness and had little money left in savings. My health insurance was hassling me, bills were piling up, and every aspect of my future was in question. I did not immediately say, "Oh, this is all an opportunity for me to grow! How wonderful! I am so grateful." To the contrary, I thought more along the lines of "If this shit doesn't end soon, I don't know how much more I can take."

I kept trying to tell myself to find the silver lining in what was happening, but all I could see was the hopelessness of it all. Then I found that if I kept trying to "be positive" without a spiritual focus, I would continue to fail.

My first step in becoming a learner was to decide, every day, that I would be one. When I began consciously making this decision each day, my health challenges began to bring wisdom to me. I came to see that there was another way to go through my illness besides feeling constantly sucker punched in the gut by life and believing there was not a damn thing I could do about it.

In order become a learner, I had to stop trying to control everything, including my body, and trust that there were lessons about Life within my situation. Even though trying to control my illness by healing the physical symptoms through medical treatment and other means appeared to be a positive thing to do, my motivation for doing so was fear; therefore, for me, trying to heal myself physically was part of a victim approach. In other words, even if my body were to get better, my experience was going to continue to stem from fear.

The learner approach is not easy, because it requires conscious intention rather than just going along for the ride of circumstance as victims do. It is much easier to feel like a victim when you're gripping the sides of the toilet bowl, puking because of the medication you're taking, or while you're getting very unwelcome news from the doctor. But it is possible to begin to adopt a learner approach to all that comes your way with a health challenge. Your task is to decide if, in all situations from now on, what you are going through can bring you something, some meaning, and then commit to finding it.

Exercise: Deciding to Be a Learner

This exercise calls you to consciously decide to move toward healing by gaining meaning from your health challenge.

I am inviting you to decide to be a learner instead of a victim. Decide with me to remember that you can find meaning in Life, even when you have been dealt a situation that appears dismal or hopeless. Decide that what matters most in dealing with your health challenge is doing your best to demonstrate your human potential at its highest. Choose to take the learner approach in order to find meaning, to discover Love, to listen to your inner teacher, to transform your health challenge into a triumph of spirit, to turn a situation that you did not want into a personal achievement that you do want. If you are facing a situation where you feel you cannot change your body or the condition, decide to challenge yourself to change yourself, to discover who you are, to embrace the Life that is within you now.

Deciding Whether to Increase Fear or the Awareness of Love

To begin becoming a learner is to begin examining our thoughts and the source(s) of our belief system. For this examination, we need to be willing to look deeply at experiences in our lives that may have contributed to fear or where we felt like a victim.

We will not bring about true healing and health if all we focus on is our physical condition and what we can do about it through medical intervention. Such an approach does not address what is at the root of our fear and, to some extent, our illness.

This is for sure: If we want to create health and have an optimum recovery, there are choices for us to make. Every day, even every hour or two, we are offered yet another opportunity to decide how we approach our lives at this very moment. This decision will determine the extent to which we allow pain, fear, worry, and anxiety to control us, rob us of our freedom, and hide our awareness of Love. This decision, which we can and may need to make often, determines whether we experience posttraumatic growth or simply become passive victims of circumstance, allowing ourselves to be molded by our physical condition rather than set free by it.

This discussion may seem lofty or impractical for someone who has so many concerns on the physical level. However, after watching many people make such a decision, I assure you that this decision is important and not a waste of your time. The cognitive and attitudinal reactions we have to facing a health challenge are much more than results or expressions of our physical condition. Even though symptoms such as pain, limited movement, and lack of energy may seem difficult to overcome, and people are bound to react in certain ways when faced with these challenges, the final analysis is always the same: *The person we become when faced with these challenges is the result of an inner decision, not the result of outside influences and our physical condition alone.* Therefore, even under the most challenging of circumstances, any of us can decide what shall become of us—even who we become as we face our mortality. *We choose our own mental and spiritual direction each and every moment.* True freedom, the basis of health, is making that choice, and the ability to make that choice is never lost to us.

Your being needs the awareness of Love like your body needs oxygen, and without the awareness of this Love, true health and vibrancy are not possible. I am not speaking here of romantic love, but of the deep spiritual Love we experience when we direct our thoughts toward Life. Have you ever wondered how someone can get older, and despite not being in physically great shape, still be vibrant, full of energy, and healthy? Think of the Dalai Lama or Mother Teresa. Is it not the Love that exudes from them that made and makes them so vibrant? This vibrant Love is the source of true health, and it is available to each of us. Any approach to healing that does not include this Love is, in my opinion, incomplete. I have witnessed the effects of this vibrant Love in many situations that were seen as hopeless, including in my own life.

I remember, for example, walking into one of Mother Teresa's Missionaries of Charity in Bombay for the first time in 1981. I expected to find misery, disease, hopelessness, and despair. But instead I found a peace and Love that were palatable. In the decades since then, I have devoted my life and work to discovering this Love, finding what blocks it, and developing ways to have it even in the most physically challenging of situations.

What I have found in myself, as well as in the many people with whom I have worked, is that some of our beliefs, thoughts, and attitudes block the natural occurrence of Love within us, and in its place emerges fear. This fear not only drains us and increases stress, but also acts as a wall to what can ultimately bring us peace of mind and true health and recovery. In my case, once I'd addressed these fear-based beliefs and thoughts, my entire experience changed. As I faced my health challenge, my work was not to only address the physical components of my condition, but to also remove my fear-based beliefs and thoughts that blocked the Love that comes naturally.

I am not saying that we should abandon the benefits of modern medicine because Love or Life is all we need to be healed. I am saying that without the awareness of Love within and around us, we will never have a vibrancy that can carry us through any health challenge in a way that brings us deeper peace and meaning.

I have seen very ill patients, and even kids with terminal cancer, with a vibrancy that comes from Love, which they did not experience until their illness. They found this Love, in part, by making the decisions discussed in this chapter. Did they all live? No. Some did, some did not. But they all experienced Love and peace beyond what they had ever known, and in many cases, so did the people around them.

If we don't reduce fear and increase our awareness of Love, our physical health does not mean much, even when we have it. I have seen many physically healthy people who are miserable. I have also seen bald-headed children facing the possibility of death discover the tremendous peace that comes from reducing fear by saying yes to Life. Which group is truly healthy: the miserable, physically sound adults or the happy sick kids? Do not make the mistake of thinking that physical health is all you need in order to be happy, or that without physical health, you cannot have the outlook and attitude that vibrant Love can bring.

As another example, think of a farmer who spends all his time looking for the best of plants, invests a lot of money and time in them, but puts very little effort into finding rich soil, good water, and plenty of sun in which to place them. If we spend time and effort only on our physical condition, we are like the farmer spending time and effort only on having good plants. We need the rich soil of the awareness of Love, the pure water of clear thinking and attitudes, and the welcome rays of that which radiates from something much larger than ourselves.

Deciding Where to Invest Time and Energy

Though I am not always perfect in my practice of removing obstacles to the awareness of Love, I have come to know the formula that leads to increased fear and the formula that leads to true health.

- ❖ If you believe your body and physical health are the primary source of your happiness, you will invest primarily in them, and you will be very fearful because your body is not very reliable over time.

- ❖ If you believe the vibrancy of Love is the primary source of your happiness, you will invest primarily in it, and you will experience growth even during a health challenge.

Visually, these two formulas look like this:

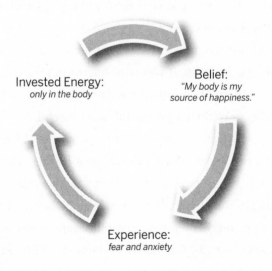

Invested Energy:
only in the body

Belief:
"My body is my source of happiness."

Experience:
fear and anxiety

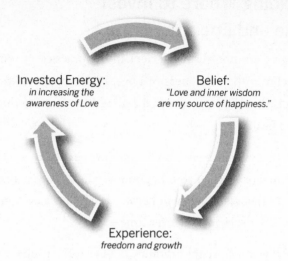

Invested Energy:
*in increasing the
awareness of Love*

Belief:
*"Love and inner wisdom
are my source of happiness."*

Experience:
freedom and growth

These are very important formulas to understand, because your beliefs about where your happiness and peace of mind come from will determine how you approach your health challenge and where you invest the most time and energy. And your approach, where you put your time and energy, will, in turn, determine your experience.

Though overcoming a disease through modern medicine certainly has benefits, if you continue to hold on to certain beliefs and thoughts, you will not discover increased purpose or meaning or become more loving and peaceful.

The most effective ways to start improving your health *and* your life are to decide that you will be a learner instead of a victim and to decide to believe and trust that no matter what is happening to you physically, you can become a more spiritually centered person. Remember, research clearly demonstrates a link between our physical health and our thoughts, emotions, and beliefs. And even the most conservative Western physician will agree that there is a power in the placebo effect, which says that what a patient believes greatly influences his or her medical outcome. Therefore, making the decision to change your mind has the power to change your health.

Deciding What to Believe and What to Value

Once there was a young boy whose father was very ill and about to die. The day before death found its way to their small cottage, the father, delirious with fever, placed some shiny stones in the boy's hand. As the boy held them in his palm, examining them closely, his father whispered with a raspy voice, "If you plant these magic stones in the earth, a tree will grow. This tree will bear fruit that will give you everything you want and need, now and always."

Although the boy was very sad about his father's illness, he was also excited by the wonderful and secret gift. The moment the boy closed his fingers around the cool stones, he believed that they were his key to finding happiness, and he valued them greatly.

The eager lad ventured out of the house and found a small plot of soil he felt would be perfect for his "seeds." With great care, he dug several small holes and planted the stones, thinking how lucky he was and how beautiful his tree would be. He was very sad that his father would not be alive see his tree when it was grown.

After his father's death, the boy visited the plot day after day, enthusiastically awaiting the first signs of growth. Each day he got down on his hands and knees, looking for a sprout, yet found nothing but the dry dirt he had left the day before.

He continued watching for sprouts for years, neglecting all other areas of his existence because he believed the stones to be of such great value. But as the boy grew older, he began to wonder why the beautiful tree his father had promised was not growing. With each passing year, he became more frustrated. He also began to feel angry at his father for not telling him more about how to make the seeds grow. But he never questioned the worth of the magic stones.

Finally, he ventured out into the world to find a solution to his predicament. Traveling down a worn cobblestone path, he came across the old gardener for the town park. "What luck!" the boy thought to himself.

Being guarded about his magic seeds, he told the old man only that he wanted to know how to grow plants, because he was trying to grow a tree from seeds his father had given him just before his death.

"What a beautiful tree it will be," the gardener responded with a kind smile. "For anything to grow well, it needs nurturing, plenty of water, and ample sun."

"Well," the young man said to himself, "that is obviously the problem. The plot of land I chose as a child was in the shade, and I had no idea how much water was needed."

As the young man made his way home, this new information depressed him because he had invested so much time in cultivating his tree. But the next day was a beautiful spring morning, and he was happy because he believed that it was simply the shady plot and lack of water that had caused his misfortune. With the rising sun, he went to his plot, dug up his stones, and carefully replanted them in a sunny spot, close to a stream where he could get plenty of water for them.

Within a few days, he began to see some growth and was exhilarated. More motivated than ever, he continued to water the small green sprouts that he saw protruding from the soil. It would be only a matter of time before his tree was in full bloom!

After a few days, the young man proudly showed the old gardener his sprouting tree, beaming with enthusiasm. The gardener, a kind person who had always been delighted to help anybody who took an interest in the earth and in plants, thought to himself, "How will I tell this young man that there is no sprouting tree, and that all this effort, water, and sunlight has produced only weeds?"

After a few moments of thought, the gardener decided that the young man would be best served by the truth. So the old man told him that his tree was still a long way from being full grown. He told the young man that if he wanted his tree to grow, he needed to pull out the weeds and clear the soil.

The young man did not welcome the gardener's advice. He was unhappy at being told he had to pull up and throw away what he had waited most of his life to see and what, only a moment ago, he had valued more than anything.

Yet the next day, the gardener found the young man pulling up the weeds, while barely holding back his tears. The gardener was most impressed that the young man had the courage to persevere many years and put in much time and effort in order to grow his father's tree. For this reason, he decided to help the young man determine the problem.

"Do you know where your father purchased his seeds, and what kind of tree you are trying to grow?" the gardener asked.

Beginning to trust the gardener, the young man hesitantly replied, "The seeds were shiny stones. My father gave them to me when I was very small. His dying words were that the tree would bear fruit that would give me everything I wanted and needed, now and always."

Now the gardener faced a dilemma. He could tell the young man that his seeds were merely everyday rocks, perhaps pretty, but they would not grow into anything. But he feared that telling the young man this would break his spirit. Conversely, if the gardener didn't tell him the truth, the young man would only go on valuing something that has no value, spending his life in endless disappointment.

In the end, the gardener again decided that the young man would be best served by knowing the truth. Perhaps with the truth, the gardener thought, the lad would be able to start life anew. The young man had isolated himself and had little contact with other people because he had been certain that other people would want his tree for themselves. And because he had believed that the tree would offer him everything, he had believed he would need nothing else.

The gardener reached down and dug in the soil where the young man had been pulling the weeds. With one hand, the gardener gathered up the stones. Then he rested his other hand on the young man's shoulder. He gently told the young man the truth.

How painful it was for the young man to hear that the tree his father had promised had existed only in the dying man's delirious mind. His magic tree would never grow.

As the young man realized he had put all his energy into something valueless, he became angry about all the time that he had wasted. More than anything, he was angry and hurt that his father had deceived him, even though he knew his father had not been in his right mind when he gave him the stones.

For a moment, the young man wondered if the gardener was really telling him the truth. He wondered if perhaps the gardener wanted the magic stones for himself. But these thoughts passed. And after a few days, the young man realized that his belief had caused him to spend his life searching for happiness in an illusion, where it would never be found.

The gardener, being a wise and learned soul, began to take long walks with the young man. He helped the young man see that though there was no magic tree, there could be something better.

He told the young man, "Much like the sun and water nourish seeds and enable them to grow something remarkable, Spirit takes the seeds of love and kindness within you and allows you to grow into something extraordinary. Spirit even uses your mistakes about looking elsewhere for happiness to help you learn about the depth of love."

The young man slowly began to want this "something better," and the two talked further about the young man's beliefs that had blocked him from having it. It was not a painless process, but for the first time, the young man stepped out of the painful existence that comes from false beliefs and into a new world of light and hope.

This parable of the young man and the gardener, adapted from one of my earlier books, illustrates how being a victim of fear affects how we experience our health challenge.

The delirious father, who gave the boy the stones and promised they would give him all he wants and needs, represents the ego, the fearful part of our mind that believes it is separate from Love, from Life, from nature, and from other people. The ego sends us looking for happiness in places we will never find it in any lasting way. The ego believes the body is who we are. The ego never looks toward any inner wisdom; in fact, it fears that inner teacher.

The stones the boy receives represent the belief that the body and physical health are the sole sources of happiness and well-being. Life (or Love, our inner teacher) is the gardener, dispelling our illusion and telling us there is something much better. The isolation the young man encounters represents how we can cut ourselves off from others and isolate ourselves when we're facing a health challenge.

The parable of the young man and the gardener is the story of much of my life. Beginning early in life, I adopted certain erroneous beliefs about where and how I would find happiness, and then I spent a good portion of my energy pursuing happiness in these places and via these means. Like the young man, I watered many weeds, thinking they would grow into what I wanted. It was through the experience of physical illness that I began to see how much I believed that my physical health and material surroundings determined my happiness, and how wrong this belief was. Sometimes it takes having the rug completely pulled out from our feet for us to see where true stability and happiness come from, and certainly my health challenges pulled the rug out from beneath me.

For the young man to be able to do something different with his life, he first needed to realize that as long as he continued to believe the stones were magic seeds, his life would never be any other way. Similarly, I needed to realize that as long as I continued to believe that being happy meant I had to be in near perfect physical health, with all my abilities and senses intact, I could not see the possibility of Life-centered living.

A strong body and physical health can be blessings, but do not make the mistake of believing that your body has to be a certain way in order for you to be happy. If you do, you will become slave to a never-ending pursuit of the ego.

CHAPTER SIX

Health-Inhibiting and Health-Enhancing Beliefs

When the drug is taken away from the addict, that person experiences pain and discomfort. This is obviously not because the removed substance is "good" for them. Rather, addicts have become so used to the drug that their bodies and minds *believe* the drug is needed and, therefore, on some level, is "good" for them.

When I was facing my health challenges, I realized that I had become addicted to my beliefs about health and the body in the same way an addict is hooked on a drug. This addiction kept me from being able to find the freedom that I desired. Even after I had identified the beliefs that continually led me into inner turmoil, I would experience deep loss and pain when I tried to give them up. For example, even after I knew that believing I needed my hearing to be happy was erroneous, trying to give up this thought did not seem to bring me any immediate peace. My mind had become addicted to thinking in certain ways and having a certain image of myself. When I tried to change, I faced great resistance, because for so long I had believed that any physical disability meant decreased happiness.

The beliefs I had unconsciously adopted had become part of a downward spiral that was anything but healthy, and all of them could be traced back to three common core health-inhibiting beliefs. But I was able to overcome the obstacles to uprooting these beliefs and replace them with three health-enhancing beliefs. In doing so, I began to live a fuller life, even though my health challenge did not change.

Three Core Health-Inhibiting Beliefs

Allan was experiencing the mixed bag of feelings that comes after a health challenge. He was two months into dealing with severe complications to diabetes. Though he was a bright man, he had never adopted a healthy lifestyle that took his disease into consideration. His diet was poor, and his exercise was limited. Further, over the time since his illness had gotten worse, he and his wife seldom communicated with one another. Most of their time was spent in front of the television. Allan felt that his life was void of any meaning but saw little possibility of anything different, physically or emotionally. He had never seriously thought of suicide, but sometimes he wondered if there were any way his life could ever be satisfying.

Allan had adopted the three core health-inhibiting beliefs:

1. Judging and criticizing ourselves, our bodies, our health, and others will lead to good health and positive change.

2. Being angry and/or worried about what is happening, has happened in the past, or might happen in the future helps us become healthy.

3. Controlling the situation will lead to health and happiness.

Most people have adopted these three core beliefs to some extent. Some sub-beliefs that contribute to fear during a health challenge can appear to have little to do with the present situation or even our physical bodies. We acquire these sub-beliefs for a variety of reasons, but there are certain commonalities between the sub-beliefs, and the beliefs do affect our health.

Let's examine the core beliefs in detail, including how and when each belief originated in Allan's life.

1. Judging and criticizing ourselves, our bodies, our health, and others will lead to good health and positive change.

It is amazing how often people either consciously or unconsciously judge and criticize themselves for being sick, old, out of shape, or otherwise not physically ideal. This self-criticism is even more pronounced if they have engaged in a behavior that contributed to their present health challenge, such as smoking or drinking.

Typical side effects of this belief include thinking you are not good enough, believing that you will never be as happy as you would like to be, believing you won't amount to what you had hoped, acting judgmental of others, and believing that true health is never going to happen for you.

In Allan's case, his father was always criticizing him, including for the fact that he was not athletic enough. No matter how well Allan performed any activity as a child, his father would tell Allan how he could have done it better.

2. Being angry and/or worried about what is happening, has happened in the past, or might happen in the future helps us become healthy.

During a health challenge, the mind wants to run wild with fear, and the form that fear often takes is anger and/or worry about the past and future, and fighting or avoiding what is happening now.

Typical side effects of this belief include acting as though being upset will keep you safer and healthier and make what is happening not happen, building defensive walls and thinking they will bring security, turning anger inward and creating more stress and disease, believing resentments build protection, and thinking that communication about what is upsetting you should be kept to a minimum.

Allan's parents coexisted with each other but never expressed any verbal or physical warmth toward each other or Allan. His family culture taught Allan that strength lay in fighting conditions we don't want.

3. Controlling the situation will lead to health and happiness.

Modern medicine is primarily about controlling. Controlling is not always a bad approach; antibiotics can control a variety of diseases, and surgery can control the spread of cancer, for example. However, when, in our minds, we approach our health challenge only from a place of control, we miss many opportunities to learn and grow from what is happening.

Typical side effects of this belief include thinking (ironically) that you don't have any control over or choices in your life, micromanaging people and situations, working too much, and experiencing high stress and stress-related disease.

Allan saw all members of his family as unhappy, unhealthy, resentful, rageful, and fearful. He concluded that they were this way because of external circumstances beyond their control. He saw their reactions as normal. He learned from society that being able to control situations was a strength and that anything short of staying in control was failure.

Exercise: Contemplating the Three Health-Inhibiting Beliefs

Please reread the descriptions of each core health-inhibiting belief. Ask yourself how each of these three beliefs shows up in your life. Then ask yourself what their origins might be.

Three Core Health-Enhancing Beliefs (and the Three Thoughts That Block Them)

During a health challenge, it is important to remind yourself quite often that the three core health-inhibiting beliefs lead to a life devoid of Love, vibrancy, and true health and happiness.

However, completely letting go of the three health-inhibiting beliefs is not always simple. I know this firsthand. Like most people, I created obstacles and fears that thwarted my early attempts at finding the ability to say yes to Life. Though determining the exact origin of the three core health-inhibiting beliefs is important, it is not as important as confronting and working through our obstacles to release them. I have met many miserable people who can talk endlessly about why they are that way. Simple insight into something does not necessarily lead to deep change and a deep commitment to inner peace.

The following three health-enhancing beliefs can replace each of the three core health-inhibiting beliefs and the obstacles that you may encounter, as I did, as you strive to embrace each one.

1. Despite my health challenge, I am capable of feeling centered and choosing peace.

Obstacle: Other people and I will see my mistakes as failures.

2. Being willing to forgive and let go will create peace of mind.

Obstacle: Forgiveness has nothing to do with health; wanting to forgive is a weakness and will make other people take advantage of me when I am most vulnerable.

3. My health challenge and current situation do not determine my experience. Other people's reactions to my illness may be about their fears; they are not about me.

Obstacle: Taking responsibility for my responses to my illness means I can no longer have an excuse in front of others or be a victim.

All these obstacles have two things in common: First, they were thoughts and beliefs, not facts. Second, they blocked my ability to learn and grow, which is to say, they blocked me from saying yes to Life.

I call all these obstacles *health-blocker thoughts*, because they are how my fear blocks me from embracing health-enhancing beliefs, and they keep me entrenched in my old way of thinking. Health-blocker thoughts illustrate the fear factor within my thinking. I have never met anyone with a health challenge who has not had some of these thoughts and needed to deal with them.

As they did with me, health-blocker thoughts have likely caused you unnecessary suffering, and they may be contributing to your illness or slowing your healing. I had to become willing to confront the dysfunctional ways I was continuing to think, and to see that these thoughts did nothing to make my life how I wanted it to be. If I had spent even a fraction of the amount of time addressing my health-blocker thoughts as I did worrying and going from one doctor's appointment to the next, I would have found health much more quickly.

Counteracting Fear, Hopelessness, and Health-Blocker Thoughts

There may well be a part of your mind telling you that making this type of change in your thinking is dangerous, perhaps even naive. When hopelessness of any kind arises in response to your health challenge, pause and say, "There is another way to see this. True health—peace of mind—is possible." I was amazed at how merely saying these words as often as possible helped turn my experience in a positive direction. I even wrote this saying down on a three-by-five card and kept it where I would see it throughout the day. Slowly I adopted an outlook in which I was no longer a victim of my health challenge and life situation.

The phrase "There is another way to see this. Health is possible," delineates two distinctly different worlds based on two different sets of values and beliefs. You are essentially saying "I am beginning to trust that beyond my ego's response to my health challenge is a world of peace and true health that is kept safe for me, where true health patiently awaits. I am choosing to set my mind in this direction."

Health-blocker thoughts scream, "Help me to be healthier, but please don't make me give up anything I think I want!" In the early stages of saying yes to Life, you may feel you are being asked to give up something useful, or you may be concerned that you will be asked to do so in later steps. Please understand that you are not being asked, nor will you be, to give up anything useful. Ask the alcoholic to give up booze, and it is unlikely you will get a positive response. Similarly, ask someone who is just beginning to deal with a health challenge to completely change their thinking and let go of fearful thoughts, and you will be met with resistance.

At this stage of developing health, your only task is to fan the spark of faith that a richer life is possible even though you have a health challenge. You do this by saying to yourself, as often as possible, "I want something better. There is another way to see my health challenge besides feeling like a victim or being afraid. Health is possible." Don't even concern yourself with believing these words right now; just practice saying them.

Exercise: Developing Positive Presence

On a sheet of paper, list all aspects of your life that are not as you would like them to be, or that you fear will become as you don't want them to be, because of your health challenge. Be specific. Don't just write, "I can't do what I used to do." Rather, describe what you can't or won't be able to do in a way that is both very detailed and illustrates your feelings. For example, you might write, "I am afraid I won't be able to work in my profession any longer."

Begin to think about the three core health-inhibiting beliefs and how they contribute to the things you don't like about your life since your health challenge began. For example, if you wrote, "I don't get enough under-standing about my condition from people around me," ask yourself, "Do I believe that I am worthwhile, or am I judging myself harshly? Am I angry about what I can't do anymore? Do I have a chip on my shoulder because I am worried and tired a lot of the time?" Even in areas of your life where you feel comfortable, list the aspects that are less than desirable. Do not rush through this list. Spend some time on it each day for about a week.

When you are looking at your life since the onset of your health challenge, you might focus on your work, your relationship with your partner (or the lack of a relationship), your relationship with your parents and/ or kids, your social life, your sexuality, your spirituality, your intellectual life, your emotional life, and your body image.

When you are all done with your lists, make a title page for your work. The title page should say:

Freedom is possible from all of what follows.

The following are the effects of my present way of thinking.

If I want to change these aspects of my life, I will need to believe that there is something better in store for me and there is another way to see my health challenge.

Then read the volume each day. It will serve as a reminder of how to direct your thoughts.

Surface Goals versus Meaningful Change: Directing the Mind to What Is Most Important

When I was not doing well physically and facing severe situations, all I could think about was getting better, getting back to life as I had known it. Quite understandably. But I found that the key to real health was not only getting well physically, but also becoming spiritually well, regardless of the state of my body. Sure, who doesn't want to be physically healthy? But given the choice of being physically healthy while being spiritually empty, and being spiritually full while being physically challenged, I would take the latter, hands down. It was important for me to see what true health was and not get sucked into the delusion that physical health was the most important thing.

I fell short of the life I wanted for straightforward reasons. I spent precious time pursuing what I call surface goals rather than developing a response to my health challenge that would bring me spiritual depth and meaning. Surface goals always have to do with what is impermanent, ranging from physical health to material wealth. Developing spiritual depth always has to do with what is everlasting, such as Life, Love, compassion, kindness, and forgiveness.

To distinguish a surface goal from deep and meaningful change, I sometimes use the metaphor of remodeling a home.

A number of years back, I decided to do some upgrading on my house. The original structure itself was quite old and was never intended for year-round use. The foundation was essentially nonexistent, and the quality of the original lumber was poor. Like most homeowners, I wanted something better, but I didn't want to spend much money.

The contractor told me if I added on to the house without addressing the core problems, I would most likely have larger problems in a few years. He suggested that I redo the whole structure—a project that required considerably more time, work, and money.

Naturally, I met this recommendation with resistance. My surface goal was to just fix up the place so it looked better from the outside and had good curb appeal. But eventually, because of the contractor's persistence, I conceded, and I am now much happier because of it. Knowing that my home doesn't just look good but is also structurally sound gives me great peace of mind.

I have come to see that only pursuing the surface goal of physical health considerably limits my potential to learn some of the most important lessons life has to offer. In our lives, surface goals usually have to do with external appearances and what we can do. They lead only to surface changes that rarely endure. In order to make any deep change, we must first truly commit to developing more trust in Life.

To acquire this depth of motivation and commitment, I needed to recognize the inherent problems with some of my beliefs. This process was an essential aspect of developing trust in myself and in Life and of coming to believe there were lessons for me to learn in my health challenge.

I resisted this process tremendously. Like the young man in the parable in the last chapter, I did not want to discover that the way I thought was dysfunctional. I was very attached to the way I thought and to my value system. I thought my physical health was of paramount importance, and my value system did not include health challenges. When I was honest with myself, I saw that when my thought, belief, and value systems were threatened in any way, I became very defensive.

Valuing Fearlessness

In 1989, Chinese students and other citizens staged a massive demonstration in Beijing's Tiananmen Square to protest oppression by their communist government. The Chinese government, no doubt fearing a new and different way of thinking, responded to that move with great violence, sending military tanks into the square to fire on the protestors. Despite the danger, some young men and women persevered in their quest for freedom. One now-legendary news photograph shows a single student standing firmly and resolutely in front of a tank, stopping it in its tracks.

It is an image that has stayed with me for years. For me, that scene is a metaphor for how to approach a health challenge. The tank represents my old beliefs about my health and how I have lived my life. The single student is my resolve to develop a better response to my health challenge and embrace health-enhancing beliefs. In dealing with my health challenges, I needed to stand in front of all of my fears and say "Stop! There is a better way! Instead of being run by my fears, I can learn to Love more deeply."

I have come to believe that if I am not experiencing peace of mind, it can only be for one reason: I continually invest time and energy in areas that repeatedly lead away from the lessons that are here right now.

CHAPTER SEVEN

Facing Our Schemas: Seven Truths to Change Our Thinking

Once we understand what true health is and what blocks it, we can embark on specific ways to overcome obstacles to our health and healing. This chapter introduces seven truths that prompt us to explore how our ego and current fear-based thinking—our schemas—keep us from true health. Within each truth is an invitation that, if we accept it, will lead us to let go of fear and say yes to Life and Love.

Truth One: What Is Everlasting Has Complete Value; What Is Impermanent Has Limited Value

This truth guides us to recognize what is valuable and what is valueless. To do this, we must first recognize the beliefs and thoughts—the schemas—that lead us to value things that are impermanent.

Each of us, at all times, has a specific view of the world and ourselves. These views are based on the various lenses through which we look—our beliefs and ways of thinking. I refer to these lenses as schemas, and I put them into two different groups. Positive schemas, because they lead us to value that which is permanent—Life and Love—lead us to healing, purpose, decreased pain, a sense of inner calm, self-esteem, and peace of mind. Negative schemas, because they tell us to over-value things that are impermanent, like our bodies and material possessions, inhibit healing and lead to increased tension, stress, fear, pain, low self-worth, unhappiness, and lack of trust. Almost all negative schemas are based on one or all of the three core health-inhibiting beliefs.

Part of developing the state of mind that leads to posttraumatic growth is acquiring the skill to determine which schemas are positive and which are negative. This may seem obvious, but schemas, being products of the ego, are often very sneaky.

One negative schema I and many others have fallen prey to in the past is what I call not-enough thinking. When we have little or no awareness and insight about the nature of impermanence, we develop, unconsciously, a condition where we secretly believe we are never enough, and that we can never have enough. I recall being entrenched in this schema when I was sick, tired, and in pain for what felt like forever. I felt that no matter what I did, I would never be healthy, have the life I once did, or be without pain. At the same time, I assumed I was totally rational and logical. But this way of thinking is hardly rational because it was based on projecting the pain and suffering I was experiencing into the future.

In our culture today, the not-enough thinking (which arises from not being aware that what is impermanent lacks value) most commonly manifests in one of three areas: *health* (feelings of losing or not having health and youth), *love* (feelings of not having enough love—the kind of love that is ego-based and seen as a commodity to get and not lose), and *money* (feelings of not having enough money and that more money would mean more happiness—despite research to the contrary).

These three areas—keeping youthful health, ego-based love, and money—are the primary gateways to confusion of value in our culture. Note the impermanent nature of each and how much happiness we believe will come from these when their pursuit actually lands us in turmoil. Intellectually seeing this is not that tough, but deeply having this shift in awareness is another story. A health challenge can wake us up to what is impermanent and the source of suffering, but it is not necessarily an easy awakening.

It is important to contemplate what is impermanent so you may see the origins of suffering. If something is impermanent, it is subject to change, and because of this, suffering can enter the scene. Much of suffering comes from the combination of denial (denying something's impermanence) and desire (desiring something that is impermanent). Realizing the nature of impermanence is liberating.

When I went to college at age eighteen, I had a very difficult time adjusting; in fact, I had never felt quite so alone. Looking back more than four decades later, I see that college was the point at which I began to experience the feeling of aloneness that I had always had but never allowed myself to feel. My way of dealing with it was to bury myself in my studies or work, a pattern that persisted for many years. When I did do something socially, I felt out of place and extremely awkward. Other people seemed to have an ease about them that I didn't have. Fear became my constant companion, and depression was close on its heels. I became convinced that I was different from others, especially socially, and that I would never be able to have "normal" relationships. I longed for acceptance and love, yet felt I was unlovable, or at least quite odd.

As the years went on, burying myself in books and work did not seem to be easing the pain. I felt that love had somehow passed me by. I began to loathe the way I was yet could find no other way of seeing myself or the world. Strangely, my only reprieve came during health challenges, when my time and energy were completely occupied. Narcotics, prescribed for pain, became my substitute for love, and to some extent my overcoming health challenges became a fragile source of esteem. (Drug addiction is the epitome of impermanence, in that we desire a state that we know will not last and become willing to sacrifice all to chase it down.) Intellectual achievement became my substitute for self-worth. I was engaged in a dangerous balancing act—seeking an impermanent state and trying to make it last—one of achievement and looking good on the outside while using drugs to numb myself on the inside.

I graduated from college in less than two years and was in graduate school at age nineteen. The elixir of achievement and drugs continued to give me a feeling of pseudo success, an impermanent imitation of what was missing in my life. But my trust of other people and Life all but vanished. The only things I trusted were the beliefs that I was never going to really be happy and healthy or have intimate and close relationships. These beliefs were built from valuing and seeking the impermanent and failing at it, yet not recognizing any of the process. I projected this failure belief into the future so well that, for a time, I became completely isolated. I had some problems with overdosing on drugs, and because of my isolation, there was nobody to save me. By valuing and seeking happiness within that which is impermanent, I had built a house of cards and lived inside of it, constantly afraid of the inevitable collapse.

Somehow, through all this, came a few glimmers of hope for something better. There was nothing specific—just a feeling of hope despite the circumstances. I truly believe that the permanence of Love finds ways to reach us even when we value the impermanent and are in overwhelming suffering because of it. I started to believe that my life could be another way, that I could have the circumstances that I was dealt *and* still find purpose and happiness. There was no particular reason for me to have this belief. Love just found ways for me to find it. Somehow, despite my physical condition, I began to believe there was Love to be discovered and shared, and that this would reduce my suffering.

At first I had no idea what I could do to change my experience. I was not thinking in terms of permanent or impermanent, no more than you have likely been. Then slowly it became clear that there was something more, something everlasting, some thread of peace in all of Life that had inherent value. I knew that to gain more insight I was going to have to turn to something larger than myself. The first step I took was praying for a different approach to my life. I didn't enter a completely vulnerable place, but those initial prayers were the beginning of my trust in Love, of finally seeing within my endless pursuit of what was valueless and impermanent. Saying yes to Life is patient and content with the smallest of efforts on our part.

Based on my personal experience and my work with many other health-challenged people, I firmly believe that *to reverse any negative schema, we only need to begin to want something other than meaningless pain and suffering, and we begin this by contemplating what is impermanent.*

Even the dimmest light in a dark room transforms the darkness. For me, believing in and valuing the small spark of Love, which is forever within me, changed my life forever. Over the years, this spark has ignited a fire in my belly, and I now am living the "something better" I once imagined. I value Love, which is all there is, has complete value, and is everlasting.

Truth Two: Suffering Is Increased by Projecting Pain into the Future

This truth guides us to recognize what really increases suffering: negative schemas that project our current pain into the future.

It is impossible to believe that healing (letting go of fear) is possible as long as we project pain and suffering into the future. Not-enough thinking, projecting our fears of not being enough or having enough into the future and thereby increasing suffering through worry and fear, is only one example of a negative schema that will lead us into increased pain and suffering.

Although the list of negative schemas that can keep us from finding true healing is endless, the following are five of the most common. After each schema is the type of suffering that results from it.

1. Pain and sickness are the worst things in life, and I should fear them. A spiritual approach to such matters is a luxury, maybe even a waste of precious time.

Fear/future projection: Sooner or later I am going to be incapacitated and in more pain. Pain and sickness are inevitable.

Resulting suffering: *I always fear aging, illness, and pain. I am on the lookout for how much I might suffer. I feel alone, angry, and afraid most of the time. I am not in touch with any spiritual aspect of my life on any consistent basis.*

2. My self-esteem and self-worth come from having a healthy body and looking good. Having visible symptoms or showing how I feel when I'm not well are signs of weakness. It is more important to keep up a good front than to let anybody see how my body is or how I feel.

Fear/future projection: My body won't always look good and be healthy. Someday I will be weak, and I will be rejected for it.

Resulting suffering: *I am preoccupied with my body. I tend to be a workaholic or have other ways of distracting myself, so I do not have to admit when I am tired or not well.*

3. I follow the adage "The one who dies with the most toys wins." More money and material possessions bring increased happiness.

Fear/future projection: I won't have enough money in the future to take care of myself.

Resulting suffering: *I never feel adequate because there is always something else—something newer or better— to acquire. I spend a lot of money on health products but don't really look much at my thinking. When I purchase something new or make more money, I experience momentary happiness, but then there is something else to get or more money to be made. I compare myself with others all the time and, as a result, vacillate between feeling superior or inferior. When I become physically ill, health becomes just a commodity.*

4. What I achieve is who I am. Beating an illness means I am a success; not doing so means I am a failure.

Fear/future projection: I am not going to be able to keep up with achieving all my goals. My condition is going to worsen, and people are going to see me as a failure.

Resulting suffering: *I am constantly chasing some sort of goal (including good health), yet when I achieve it, I receive only momentary satisfaction, if that. If I am not in control or in the process of achieving a new goal, I don't feel very safe or secure. Illness is the epitome of not being in control, and it makes happiness impossible.*

5. I am a victim of the world. More bad things will happen if I am not constantly on the defensive.

Fear/future projection: Nothing is going to go right, no matter how hard I try.

Resulting suffering: *I feel as though the world is against me, and my illness is proof that it is. If there is a power greater than me, it is not looking out for me. I feel like a victim. I have no power or choice in my life, and I am angry, jealous, and resentful. If I'm not careful, I tend to be a chronic blamer. I feel that things just happen to me. I have no control over my life, and I take no responsibility for my life.*

Truth Three: Love Is a Power Greater Than Your Ego, and It Is Available to You Now

This truth guides us to believe in Love, no matter our physical condition, and to remember that if we want Love to help us find purpose in what is happening in our lives, we must first learn how we use negative schemas. Though Love is available to us at any time, we need to learn how to access it by recognizing how the ego is very skilled at distracting us from it with negative schemas.

When you first begin dealing with your health challenge, it is not important to identify and analyze all your schemas. It is more important to know that they stem from the three core health-inhibiting beliefs. It is also important to begin recognizing that whenever you are suffering in any way, there is another way of looking at your illness and pain: through the power within—Love.

Though you may not yet be ready admit it, how much you suffer reflects how unwilling you are to release old ways of thinking. Please don't take offense at this statement. I say it because I know this unwillingness well myself, having spent much of my life experiencing its unfortunate effects. When my mind was arrogantly turning away from Love and any higher purpose, the statement "There is another way of looking at my illness and pain" meant nothing. In fact, I thought such a statement naive, if not laughable. My closed and untrusting mind said, "There is only one way to see my health challenge: It should not be happening, and I must to do everything I can to make it stop." Your thinking determines the degree to which you are able to turn to Love during a health challenge and, thus, the degree to which you are able to learn and grow from what is happening.

If we want to discover true healing, we must work with our thoughts. We must fully accept and embrace the simple statement "Our thoughts create." Only then are we able to understand how our health challenge can become our teacher and take responsibility for our own healing.

If you want to discover what lessons are within your health challenge, you must be willing to increasingly turn within, trusting in some way that Life and Love are within you now—tender, kind, and healing. Your awareness of Love, or lack of it, determines how you remember something that happened in the past, how you see something that is happening now, and how you will see it in the future.

In the past, when I viewed my health in a black-and-white way, I believed that my negative self-image and my image of what my future held were accurate. I failed to see that I had a distorted view of what was happening to me, based on my ego's negative schemas, and that I had no awareness of my inner wisdom. As a result, I carried around the weight of emotional upset and physical pain.

In order to heal my thinking, I had to be willing to

- own what I was afraid of instead of projecting it into the future, and

- ask my inner wisdom (Love) what lessons I could learn from what was happening.

To find true healing during a serious health challenge, we must do the deeper work of looking into our inner lives, how we see ourselves, and how we see the world. Fortunately, we can do this work along with any medical treatment we may be receiving now or in the future.

The experiences we had when we were growing up contribute to our distorted perception of ourselves, which then has an impact on our health and healing. Often, others tell us things about us that are far from the truth of who we really are, and we carry around the resulting negative feelings about those things for years. These negative schemas and thoughts cause stress and blocks to full healing.

It is not uncommon for old memories to emerge during a health challenge, just as the following one did for me.

When I was a sophomore in high school, I wanted to switch to a different school, and my parents agreed. My freshman year at my first school had been difficult for me socially and academically. I had been in and out of hospitals and body casts during my freshman year and had felt depressed, embarrassed, and separate from my peers. So I looked forward to being in a different environment. About halfway through my sophomore year, my parents decided to divorce. And as typically happens in alcoholic homes, nobody talked about the divorce; it was as if it had not even happened. Feeling that I couldn't talk about it, I repressed a lot of the feelings I had about the divorce. In retrospect, I had tried to keep my parents together for years before the divorce by keeping their attention focused on me. I faked accidents and illness in desperate attempts to keep them together, although at the time I wasn't conscious of the reasons behind my behavior. Hospitals and casts resulted. I was caught in a strange downward cycle, confused as to which of my health conditions were real and which were feigned.

The new school I was attending emphasized extracurricular activities, and students' academic performance was expected to be high. But I was so preoccupied with my emotional and physical situation, and I felt like such a failure coming into the school, that I rarely did any of my schoolwork and my involvement with after-school activities was minimal. I dreaded going to my classes because I knew that I would feel dumb and ashamed. Being in a body cast (still) did not help.

The inner pain I was experiencing remained locked inside and only seemed to get worse as the year progressed. Paradoxically, school was more comfortable than home. Slowly, school became a place where I felt I could be around others without the stress of conflict. I never really talked to any of the teachers, but I did feel that some understood my hidden pain, which was comforting.

At the end of the school year, I was called into the headmaster's office and told that I was being expelled. I was shocked. I was told I was not welcome back because I "was not the caliber of student or person that they wanted." The school officials added that they attributed my behavior and lack of abilities to my dealing drugs on campus. I had never dealt drugs, and the suggestion only added to my overall feeling of being judged and misunderstood, not to mention feeling alone. At the time, I had a terrible temper because of my repressed feelings and all I had been going through. In response to my expulsion, I yelled at the school officials, slammed the door as I left, and screeched off in my car, certainly confirming (at least in their eyes) that they had made the right decision.

For many years, this high school experience deeply affected me. I adopted the headmaster's assessment and really thought that I was not very intelligent or worthwhile. I never did very well the rest of high school, no doubt because I was not in class all that often. Eventually I did get involved in drugs, becoming addicted to painkillers, and my self-worth continued to decrease. My potential as a human being remained hidden from me, and probably from most other people, for many years.

It was not until I remembered this experience during a health challenge that a different awareness fully took root and became the foundation of my healing. Because my high school experience contributed a limited view of myself, it blocked full healing on any level.

As an adult facing health challenges, I have chosen to ask Love for help in changing the belief about myself that was created by this high school experience, as well as other past-based perceptions of myself. I remind myself of the following often:

- ◈ There is another way of seeing this situation.

- ◈ Believing I am anything other than worthwhile and whole indicates that I am believing in a false perception of myself rather than recognizing the Love within me.

- ◈ Never believe another person's opinion of yourself over the truth about who you are. Never believe your health challenges define who you are.

This personal story illustrates how past experiences and others' views of us contribute to our distorted perceptions of ourselves, which then impact our healing. Because I believed in the head-master's negative schema about myself, for years I was not able to see that Love is more powerful than the ego and available immediately to me. Remember, even though Love is available, it does not mean we can see it if we are being severely distracted. The invitation to believe in Love is quiet and patient, but we must turn in it's direction and choose to listen. With drugs and the loud chatter of my ego, I could not hear the gentle and quiet invitation to believe in Love. It was only by gaining the aware-ness of how I used negative schemas that I allowed Love to help me find purpose and meaning. Without this, I would not be writing these words to you at this time.

One thing I have seen repeatedly in working with people on their healing is that Love remains unharmed by what we believe about ourselves and our condition. Even in times when you believe you are alone, or you are not able to see any purpose in your situation, Love is always within you, and you will be able to see evidence of it if you look closely. In working for many years in the addiction field, I had the opportunity to see this miracle in action time and time again. I have never—not once—seen someone enter an addiction program feeling good about themselves or their behavior. Quite the contrary. Many individuals would say upon completion of the program something like "I came in here feeling like scum, and I am leaving actually feeling love and compassion for myself." Even when we believe we have not done one good deed in many years, Love patiently waits for us. We can begin today, no matter our condition, to act kindly. In my previous book, *Healing the Addictive Personality*, I go into this in great depth.

Truth Four: Life-Centered Thinking (Love) Is the Foundation of Health

This truth guides us to understand and appreciate the difference between fear-based thinking and Life-centered thinking.

We always have two mind-sets to choose from: fear-based thinking and Life-centered thinking. Each of these mind-sets has its own distinct logic and view of cause and effect.

Fear-based thinking, as the name implies, is founded on all our fears of what is happening now and what might happen down the road. This mind-set constantly searches for past, current, and future experiences to reinforce its fearful perspective. During a health challenge, the following ten core thoughts of fear-based thinking are at work:

1. Fear is real.

2. Fear of what will happen and guilt are good motivations to get better and not give up.

3. The negative aspects of my illness will likely repeat and get worse, so they should be resisted.

4. The future should be worried about and controlled.

5. I am fundamentally alone, and nobody really understands how I feel.

6. Being defensive or angry creates safety.

7. Figuring out all that is wrong will make me healthy.

8. Comparing myself to healthy people is helpful.

9. It is important for me to always be right and know what to do.

10. Blaming other people will make me feel better.

In contrast, Life-centered thinking is based on knowing that we are much more than our bodies and that love and compassion are the most healing of all forces. Life-centered thinking recognizes the interconnectedness of all life and the lessons that abound in every situation. It is the source of kindness, empathy, healing, and understanding. There are ten core thoughts of Life-centered thinking that can be at play during a health challenge, if we choose:

1. Love is the core of who I am, and Love is not dependent upon the condition of my body.

2. Forgiveness, letting go of grievances, is a central part of healing.

3. Being completely in the present moment brings renewed energy.

4. I can always choose to learn and grow from a health challenge.

5. I am, always, a part of all Life.

6. Extending compassion is always possible and always results in reducing suffering.

7. Accepting "what is" leads to peace of mind.

8. Seeing the Love we all share creates healing and wellness.

9. Turning to my inner wisdom is important.

10. I am responsible for how I react to a health challenge and what I teach.

None of our circumstances, including our health challenges, determine our inner experience. No matter what the circumstances, we are still responsible for our reactions and our peace of mind. We may not have consciously chosen our physical challenge, but we, and nobody else, are responsible for each and every thought that we have in response to it. We are not robotic computers that have no choice but to react as we're programmed. Our reactions and what we experience depend only on whether we are utilizing fear-based thinking or Life-centered thinking.

When you are having a challenging time with a particular person or health situation and decide to say "I can choose a different perception of this and a different way to respond," you are directing your mind to shift from fear-based thinking to Life-centered thinking. Commitment to this shift is necessary to heal yourself and achieve consistent peace of mind, for the two forms of thinking cannot coexist. From one comes a health challenge likely filled with suffering; from the other comes the discovery of freedom.

For many years, I was a person whose life, from an external perspective, was in order. I had a good job and just the "right" amount of material possessions. I had the word *doctor* before my name. I did not live beyond my means. I had a wife, and we had many friends. Despite all this, even before many of my health challenges, I knew deep down that I had been unhappy and confused most of my life, and that I still was.

Growing up in an alcoholic and workaholic home, I had little parental support. I was the youngest of two children and became the child with the health issues. Because of many of my health challenges, I needed continuous care and energy, though on the inside, I felt overlooked and misunderstood. I was never particularly bad or exceedingly talented at anything. Until college, I always felt that I was average or below and never stood out in any way. All my health challenges and hospitalizations gave me a way to disappear in plain sight, especially in the haze of the drugs that were administered to me.

As an adult, as I said yes to Life and Love during my health challenges, I discovered that I had lived much of my life in fear. For as long as I could remember, I had always had a deep feeling of aloneness within me. Even when I was with friends, there was still a part of me that felt alone. I found that I had always felt lacking in esteem and, in fact, often wanted to apologize for my condition, even my very existence. In all my relationships, I felt very self-conscious. I believed that I was better off keeping people at a certain distance, and I had many ways of doing so. I was a master at hiding while not looking like I was.

By developing my ability to choose Life-centered thinking, I now have more peace of mind than ever. Surprisingly, I now humbly see myself as a person who has a lot to offer the world— I believe each and every person does. I, like you, am valuable and have a core of Love. My existence matters, regardless of my body's symptoms or how long I may be alive. In short, by determining that Life-centered thinking has value and fear-based thinking does not, I have been able to mostly overcome the sense of aloneness, isolation, and mediocrity that had been with me throughout my life. And my health challenge was what motivated me to choose the Life-centered thinking mind-set. For whatever reason, when our bodies say no, it can be a time to say yes to Life and Life-centered thinking.

Truth Five: Your Ego's Way Hasn't Worked

This truth guides us to recognize that our ego's way of facing health challenges hasn't brought us health, success, or happiness.

During a health challenge, the ego diverts our attempts at Life-centered thinking by directing our mind to evaluate, compare, judge, criticize, project, condemn, hate, manipulate, shame, blame, worry, and instill guilt. Before we can let go of fear and discover full healing, we must recognize that the ego's means *never* bring us the wellness we want and keep us from healing.

When the ego sees it is losing ground to Life-centered thinking, it will sometimes try to convince us that aspects of its ways should be retained. The ego will make claims such as "In this situation, you'd better rely on anger; this all happened because you were hit by a drunk driver," or "You'll never be able to be healthy again. The odds are against recovering from this kind of cancer."

Having goals can be a pretty good thing, but having conflicting or contrary goals does not work so well. Creating conflicting goals is the ego's specialty. It asks, "Why would you want healing if you had to give up what you think is important?" We cannot successfully heal when we want both what the ego offers and all that Life-centered thinking offers. Trying to engage in Life-centered thinking while still placing value on the ego and fear-based thinking will result in constant frustration.

The truth that the ego never brings us what we want is reinforced when we examine some of the occasions we have turned to the ego for guidance. By doing this, we begin to see that *there is no value in what the ego offers,* and we can move closer to saying yes to Life.

Exercise: Choosing between the Ego and Life

This exercise is important, because until you choose between ego/fear-based thinking and Life/Life-centered thinking, it will be difficult for you to fully undertake a path toward full healing. Please give yourself plenty of time to complete the entire exercise.

On separate sheets of paper, create the following five lists. For clarification, I have included, in italics, an example of what I might include on each list if I were doing this exercise.

1. List at least ten times in your life when you have thought the condition, age, or appearance of your body determined your happiness. Include any similar thoughts you currently hold.

Example: *When I faced prostate surgery and the possibility of impotence, I believed who I was as a man was being threatened.*

2. List at least ten times when, during health challenges, large or small, you became upset or thought of yourself as inferior, unforgivable, unlovable, or something similar.

Example: *Years ago, during my initial hearing loss, I thought I would be inferior to those with hearing and incapable of having normal relationships.*

3. List at least five ways that you are now or have been afraid of the future because of a health challenge.

Example: *I have sometimes been afraid I wouldn't have enough money because of the impact of my health challenge on my career.*

4. List at least five times you became angry or defensive with someone close to you when you were actually upset about your health challenge.

Example: *I became irritable with my kids when I could not hear them because I was deaf.*

5. List at least five occasions when you have felt shame or embarrassment because of your physical condition, health challenge, or appearance.

Example: *During one hospital stay, I could no longer control my bodily functions, and someone else had to clean up the messes.*

Now go back over all of your work, asking yourself these two questions:

1. Have any of these ways of thinking or any of these actions ever resulted in peace of mind, increased and lasting healing, positive relationships, or increased awareness of Love?

2. Is there another way to think or react as I go through a health challenge?

After fully answering these questions, go back to the ten core thoughts of Life-centered thinking during a health challenge, listed on pages 105–106. Now rethink each and every situation you wrote about and ask yourself what would have occurred if you had applied these ten core thoughts at the time.

After doing this exercise, write the following on a card and spend a few days frequently reminding yourself of it:

The way of my ego and fear-based thinking increases suffering.

Life-centered thinking heals and reduces suffering.

Which I choose is up to me.

Truth Six: Through Love, Fear-Based Thinking Is Removed, and Meaning and Purpose Are Revealed

This truth guides us to overcome our primary obstacles to Life-centered thinking and, thus, our obstacles to healing.

Once we have recognized how the ego has not brought us anything other than continued suffering, we can more readily see the value of Life-centered thinking. And once we see its value, we begin to make changes that reflect true health and healing.

There have been various times in dealing with my health challenges when I needed to make important decisions. In the early 1990s, I was not able to continue working as a clinician because of my hearing loss. Some days it seemed that in any other future work I would not be doing what I really wanted to do, and I felt I was no longer making any real difference in people's lives.

My solution was to begin to write more. I began to want to do so, but my ego and fear-based thinking led me down an old, well-worn path of believing I couldn't really succeed as a writer and that I had been stripped of the only thing I was ever any good at—being a psychologist. I was clearly not believing in what was possible despite my hearing loss, and I was allowing myself to avoid dealing with what I now see as the five primary fears, or health-blocker thoughts. Each of these fears, or the avoidance of them, kept me away from Life-centered thinking.

I had a similar experience when I wanted to do more public speaking, specifically keynote presentations. I would be speaking to many thousands of people a year, in many different locations, and I was self-conscious because I could not hear people in order to converse with them or even answer questions. Below are some of the health-blocker thoughts I had in connection with my health challenge and physical limitations that arose from it. To be motivated to go beyond these fears, it was necessary for me to believe in the power of Life-centered thinking. The primary fear is in boldface type and a personal example follows. As you read them, ask yourself how these fears might be showing up in your own life, as you deal with your own health challenge.

The Fear of Failure

Example: I feared my health would continue to get worse, and that this worsening would be a sign of failure. Also, I feared that not finding career success would prove my secret belief to be true: Because of my health condition, I was now less than whole and flawed in some fundamental way.

The Fear of What Others Think

Example: I believed that when I was physically healthy, I was seen as strong. When I dealt with large hearing aids, a service dog, and not being able to hear at all, I became very self-conscious and even isolated myself from others.

The Fear of Vulnerabilities and Insecurities Being Revealed

Example: Though I don't really like to admit it, I was never all that secure. I had been hiding behind the mask of the prestige of my position as a psychologist, and I feared having to be just plain ol' Lee, especially if you threw the word *deaf* into the mix. My illness showed me that I still didn't feel fully confident in myself, and I did not want others to see how deep this insecurity went.

The Fear of "the Facts"

Example: I looked around and saw not-too-rosy health news for me on the horizon. I feared what would be in store for me. I didn't spend much time looking at all the examples of people who found posttraumatic growth in their health challenges, because I was trapped in fear-based thinking, which always looks for what will reinforce fear rather than dispel it.

The Fear That Health Conditions Are Permanent and Always Negative

Example: I projected my fears about my health so far into the future that I thought, "After all this happens to me, I will either be dead or never able to get another job. And what woman would want to be with me?"

The more I trust in the unfolding of my life and my spiritual path, the more I see that my health, healing, and success are about consciously challenging and moving beyond fears and fear-based thinking. When I am feeling tired, ill, or stressed, my ability to engage in Life-centered thinking may falter, but it is always what brings me back on track. If I am attuned to wanting healing through the spiritual practice of increasing my awareness of Love—and if I believe I can truly live a life of balance through even the darkest of times—then this healing and this life are exactly what I will create for myself.

If you find yourself fearful of making some change, work through the fear. Ask for help from the Love that is within you, even if you don't really believe you will get it. To overcome health-blocker thoughts is to remove the obstacles to Life-centered thinking. Fear-based thinking and the resulting health-blocker thoughts are like a cement wall with barbed wire atop, keeping you from being able to fully find the silver lining in your health challenges. As you begin to move through and beyond your fear and to want what Life-centered thinking offers, trust that the awareness of Love will increase in your life. The once-insurmountable walls to healing and peace of mind will then be transformed into nothing more than a rickety old fence that you can easily step over. What is truly beautiful is what can happen next, once we step over our old self-imposed walls and limitations: We discover meaning and purpose. The very book you hold in your hands at this moment came from this process. Through my own health challenges and saying yes to Life, a purpose of helping others through similar challenges was revealed.

Truth Seven: Align Your Thoughts with Love, and Healing Happens

This truth guides us to align our thoughts with Love.

After we begin to see and overcome the obstacles to Life-centered thinking, it is time for us to more fully implement the power of thought for healing, health, and wellness. This important step can quickly be discounted when our body is suffering illness and we have medical needs.

Imagine yourself sitting by a stream that is partially dammed by debris. Once you remove what is blocking the flow of water, a much stronger stream begins to pass in front of you, rushing over obstacles that were once too large for it to pass. This is what happens when we realize the power of our own thoughts to remove the debris of old thinking and support our health and healing.

However, I believe our thoughts by themselves tap only a very small part of the strength available to us. Picture yourself sitting by the ocean, rather than just a stream, contemplating the vast power of the sea and the movements of the tidal waters over the expanse of thousands of miles. If a just a small stream of thought, when undammed, can overcome obstacles, imagine what the vast strength of the ocean waters can do. The ocean is a closer representation of the strength of Love available to us in any health challenge. When we align our thoughts with Love, we are aligning ourselves with that strength in order to find purpose and meaning.

Pete was a patient I saw many years ago. He originally came to see me after completing a drug treatment program; he had become addicted to pain medication given to him for a chronic back problem over the years. Pete wanted to stay clean and sober and, in his prior attempts, had not been able to do so. He also wanted to learn alternative ways of managing his pain, which was a result of a severe auto accident.

Many of the principles of Life-centered thinking simply did not make sense to Pete. At age fifty-three, Pete had been extremely successful in his career as a research chemist with his own pharmaceutical company, and being trained as a scientist had limited him in some important ways; subjective spiritual experience, for example, made very little sense to him. If something could not be objectively quantified, he was not interested in it and had a difficult time believing it existed. He put Love in this category. Thus, when it came to realizing the power his thoughts had when aligned with Love, you might as well have been talking about an invisible fairy. Since his thoughts, let alone Love, could not be directly measured, he did not see how changing his thinking could make a difference in his life or his level of pain.

When he first came to see me, his identity was tied to his company's success, his money, and his long list of awards and publications. His thoughts seemed of little importance to him, and reducing his pain and getting off drugs were something he wanted but did not really believe to be possible. He approached life as a series of problems to solve and conquer, and his health challenge and pain were just two more of them.

During the first months that I saw Pete, he made some very profound changes in his thinking. As a result, he was able to stay off of the medication and experience some growth in other areas of his life.

However, one day, following weeks of visible progress, Pete seemed to methodically revert to his old patterns. Though he did not return to using drugs, he returned to being angry about his physical condition and felt very much like a victim. He wanted his high-achieving life back but did not see how he could get it, given all his pain and other problems from the accident. He gave up his goal of choosing to find lessons in what was happening and reverted to his objective and scientific mind.

Rather than fight all of this, I began to enter his objectified world to see if change could occur at that level. Pete was obviously under great stress because of the pain. I asked him if he would be interested in being hooked up to biofeedback machines—devices that visually depict your less conscious physiological responses. I explained that they would graphically demonstrate his heart rate, blood pressure, galvanic skin response, and brainwave pattern. I wanted to help Pete see, in objective terms that appealed to his scientific mind, that his thoughts did have a direct effect on his ability to relax, reduce pain, and be happy.

As a scientist, the idea of being able to *see* the effects of his thoughts fascinated him. Once connected to the machines, he saw that his thoughts and way of thinking were, in fact, causing objective physiological responses, including increased pain. The data painted a picture of an individual under enormous strain.

He saw how the biofeedback instruments were objectifying the results of his thinking.

With Pete's permission, I invited in a colleague who had practiced meditation for years. She also had injuries sustained in an accident and was now in a wheelchair, with a condition that typically caused her tremendous pain. She was connected to the same biofeedback machines Pete had been. I asked her to think about all the upsetting things that she could: to consciously force herself to worry about the challenges that would be in store for her physically and to think about how painful her condition could be. The machines illustrated a very stressed person.

Then I asked her to enter a meditative state, ask her inner wisdom to help lift the burden she was feeling, and even find ways to extend loving thoughts to people in that very moment. (I knew she had years of practice doing these things.) In short order, Pete saw tangible evidence of the power of a mind directed toward Life-centered thinking. For the first time, I saw in Pete's eyes that he wanted *something better* for himself and believed it was possible.

The work Pete did in therapy was far beyond what he had imagined it would be. When he started, he believed that all he needed to do to make his life a happy one was not to use pain medicine anymore and to lessen his pain in other ways. By the end, Pete had discovered the power and strength available to him when he aligned his thoughts with Love.

PART II

The Six Steps of Saying Yes

CHAPTER EIGHT

Step One: Finding a Better Way

> Things turn out the best for the people who
> make the best of the way things turn out.
>
> *John Wooden*

It is now time to make decisions about what thoughts are or aren't helpful when it comes to the pursuit of health.

Most people don't think about sorting out their thoughts when they are struggling with a health challenge, because they are so busy attending to the physical condition, with all its constant changes and demands.

Making Life-Centered Decisions

When dealing with a health challenge, we are usually called on to make many very important decisions. Some of these decisions are, quite literally, a matter of life and death. Learning how to make such decisions based on Life-centered thinking is an important aspect of saying yes to Life during a health challenge.

Eight Common Fears That Thwart Life-Centered Decision-Making

When we ask, "Did I make a good decision?" what means are we using to come to a conclusion? The fear-based and Life-centered decisions come from two very different mind-sets.

Some of your greatest advances you have judged as fail-ures, and some of your deepest retreats you have evalu-ated as success.

from A Course in Miracles

The ego—the part of our mind that is fear-based and denies Life-centered thinking—is always busy defining and analyzing. Despite the fact that the decision-making process of the ego runs off of fear and generates more fear, the ego makes decisions and then convinces us that these decisions are sound and rational.

All ego-made decisions are rooted in one or more of the following eight fears:

1. **Fear of loss (rather than knowing that happiness is an inside job)**

On one occasion I was terrified of losing what little hearing I had left. I decided to undergo a treatment that had little chance of success and the potential for side effects. Because of my fear of loss, I was not thinking clearly, and opted for this treatment. The outcome was my hearing continued to worsen, and I also suffered the severe side effects of the treatment.

2. **Fear of being inadequate (rather than trusting your inner wisdom)**

Coming from a family of doctors, I thought if I made a decision based on my intuition or decided to use any alternative medicine, I would be seen as flaky or inadequate.

3. **Fear of the future and/or time restrictions (rather than trusting the now)**

Dealing with my health challenges meant sometimes being under the gun time-wise. I believed that not reacting properly and efficiently could be catastrophic. Though having an awareness of time may be a good thing, operating from fear of it is not.

4. **Fear of abandonment (rather than knowing Love never leaves us)**

I believed if I did not get better, things might get so hard and ugly over the long haul that people would not want to be in my presence.

5. **Fear of anger (rather than knowing we can stay centered emotionally)**

I was afraid certain decisions might make somebody angry, including myself.

6. **Fear of losing power or prestige (rather than recognizing what is truly important)**

I had worked hard to get where I was in my career, and though I don't like to admit it, I feared that if I did not get well, I might have to give up some of the prestige and power that I had worked to get.

7. **Fear of embarrassment, based on feelings of shame (rather than knowing that who we are is complete and whole)**

I went through a period when I was ashamed of my physical condition; this shame certainly clouded my decision-making and isolated me from others.

8. **Fear of the body (rather than knowing that the essence of who we are is Love)**

> There were many times I was not sure I had the ability to deal with what my body was dishing out or to follow through in the ways I wanted.

For me and, I believe, for most people, making decisions based on these eight fears allowed my ego to convince me that fear-based thinking works, even though this schema actually reinforces fear and limits health and healing. As long as I made decisions based on these fears, I misguidedly thought that the ego's approach, which includes judging, analyzing, comparing, critiquing, contrasting, avoiding, controlling, attacking, competing, and intimidating, would result in decisions that would lead to positive outcomes. But what I finally realized is that decisions from these eight fears never leave me feeling safe and secure, and they certainly don't lead to health.

Seven Core Principles for Making Life-Centered Decisions

Life-centered thinking approaches decision-making from an entirely different angle than the ego; instead of making decisions based on the eight fears, Life-centered thinking bases decisions on trust in our inner wisdom and the knowledge that there are lessons to be learned in each and every moment.

Peace of mind is the highest goal of Life-centered thinking. Thus, it is best if all decisions are based on the intention to create a calm and tranquil mind.

Why is maintaining our peace of mind so important during a health challenge? As explained in chapter one, many prominent researchers are finding a direct relationship between our state of mind and our health. For example, research at Stanford University demonstrates that gaining peace of mind (by way of forgiveness) leads to increased physical vitality, hope, greater self-efficacy, and enhanced optimism. Additional research suggests that with a tranquil mind, we physiologically send messages to our bodies that allow healing to occur.

This last point is very important. Many people, especially in the worlds of medicine, business, and politics, think that spirituality—that is, focusing on peace of mind—has little significance. Nothing is further from the truth.

About twenty years ago, I had a patient, Charlie, who came to me following a very serious suicide attempt. Charlie believed his money problems and deteriorating health from diabetes would never change. He had driven his car into a tree at more than eighty miles per hour, with every intention of ending his life. But the tree he had chosen had been dead for some time, and, amazingly, it just exploded when Charlie's car hit it, causing him no life-threatening damage.

Charlie and I worked together for a little more than a year, and during that time, though his diabetes still affected his life, his *response* to his illness completely shifted. He began volunteering, fund-raising, and working with the American Diabetes Association and found that he was a surprisingly creative and effective fund-raiser. I lost contact with him for about ten years, then recently ran into him. He had his lovely wife and two teenage children with him, and I later found out he was a millionaire many times over.

"You know," he told me, "I may not be the smartest guy—I don't even have a high school education—but I now know how to ask for opportunity in my life. The only decision I really make anymore is between my old way of thinking, where I did not believe I had any opportunity in life, and my new way of thinking, where I always ask for opportunity with sincerity. All I do every day is ask Life to give me opportunity, and I humbly ask for the strength and courage to make the most of what Life brings, even when it looks like more of a challenge than an opportunity. Then, I have gratitude, and I ask Life for more opportunity. At first I thought I was greedy, always asking for more opportunity, but now I think I am just grateful and humble.

"The amazing thing is, Life just keeps giving me more opportunity. I use to think my illness was a curse; now I see it as a gift in all it taught me. I would never be where I am now without what happened. I now happily employ hundreds of people in five states, and I try to teach them the same thing that I have learned. Before, I probably would not have acted on most of the opportunities that came my way, partly because they did not always look like the opportunity I asked for. Now, I just happily work hard at doing the best I can with each opportunity Life sends my way. What other decisions are there?"

Charlie reminded me of a key truth about Life-centered decision-making:

When peace of mind and looking for opportunity in every situation are our single goal, all decisions become a means of reaching this goal.

When we are committed to Life-centered thinking, the following seven ideas will guide our decision-making:

1. **Giving and receiving are two sides of the same coin. What is truly important cannot be lost in a health challenge, and all that is of value can only increase when shared.**

Regardless of the condition of our bodies, giving and receiving love can be our central goal and focus. When I was recovering from a severe bacterial infection that took me close to death, I found that I was able to receive the love and care of those around me much more than I had in the past. Previously, giving to others had been easier for me than receiving from others, and I discovered that *with a balance of giving and receiving, we are healed.*

2. **Regardless of my physical condition, I am a whole, complete, and loving person. If I choose, my health challenge can teach me lessons that will bring more, never less, into my life.**

I have always tried to stay in shape, and I have done many athletic endeavors. At one point, my body became ravaged from my disease, and my physical ability became a shadow of what it once was. Instead of riding a bike one hundred miles, I was barely able to walk, and I was skinnier than I had ever thought I could be. It was during this time that I was guided to begin the ultimate endeavor: choosing to find the truth of who I am beyond my physical form. Now, I still strive to be in shape, but I never lose sight of the ultimate lesson: *I am not a body. I am free. I am as Life created me.*

3. **The present moment always offers the choice: Do I want what peace of mind offers, or do I want what fear offers?**

After getting repeated bad news from doctors, I found it was not easy to remain peaceful. I was afraid, no question about it. Yet at some point, I began to look at the fear, to question its origins. I said to myself, "Okay, I am afraid. This is all happening. But I don't have to take my fear as gospel. There is a quieter voice in me that says with certainty *'None of this really has an effect on the truth of who you are. None of this has the ability to stop you from giving and receiving love.'*"

4. **Through compassion for all life, my suffering is reduced.**

As I took the primary focus off of myself and my body and focused instead on extending compassion, quite miraculous things happened. *Extending compassion, rather than expending energy on suffering and preoccupation with the body, creates healing.*

5. **True health comes from the ability to love yourself and others unconditionally, regardless of the obstacles you see.**

As I stopped thinking that my health was defined by my physical state and began to see beyond all the obstacles I believed existed because of my health challenge, I found much more peace of mind. *To be healthy is to be unwavering in our commitment to seeing the opportunity to love each and every moment.*

6. **Your inner teacher, the quiet voice within, goes beyond all guilt and shame and whispers the truth. You need only to choose to listen.**

I now know that there are two distinctly different voices that I can listen to when approaching my health and physical condition: the voice of my ego or the voice of Life. *As we turn to Life, our inner teacher, we are better able to respond to what is happening now and better able to see the path ahead.*

7. **No physical condition can stop you from making gains on your spiritual path.**

I found that everything can be fodder for my spiritual growth, and within this truth, *we can live a life of gratitude rather than worrying about what may or may not happen.*

Though at times I still get trapped in the ego's fear-based way of making decisions, I have committed myself to Life-centered decision-making. So I consistently practice quieting the endless chatter of the ego and its fear-based thinking in order to allow myself to hear the wisdom of Life.

Making Decisions Based on the Power of Love

Decisions that lead to upset are characterized by the statement "I have to." Life-centered decisions are characterized by the statement "I choose to." Making decisions from an "I have to" context means primarily focusing on doing or taking some sort of action, whereas making decisions from an "I choose to" context means primarily focusing on our Life-centered attitude and secondarily focusing on action. "I choose to" decisions put the horse (Life-centered thinking) in front of the cart (our action).

Whenever we fear making a decision, we are in an "I have to" context, and we don't trust that we can find peace of mind. Here, we erroneously see our inner experience as being determined by what is happening to us and what we are doing rather than by our conscious choice and the conscious direction of our thoughts and attitude. Because of this fear and lack of trust, we can go through life without ever making any clear and committed choices—much less Life-centered decisions. Decision-making in an "I have to" context leads to passive decisions that don't serve us. It can also lead us to let other people make our decisions, form our opinions, and guide our lives. Even if we are making our own "I have to" decisions, we can internally get to the point where life appears to "just happen" to us, and we seem to be just along for the ride.

Passive decisions are decisions made without our conscious or direct choice, because we don't trust our inner wisdom or the power of Love that is always available to us. Passive decision-making is pervasive in our culture, especially in health care. People suffer because they make passive decisions and aren't committed to the healing power of Love and its direction.

Transforming an "I have to" context into an "I choose to focus on the power of Love within me" context can change everything about our decision-making experience. Following the seven core principles for making Life-centered decisions allows a richness and depth to enter into your life, and this richness and depth can be positively contagious.

Life-Centered Sharing and Relating

Along with leading me to make Life-centered decisions, saying yes to Life prompted me to start sharing more of how I was feeling on an emotional level—sometimes with other people, sometimes just acknowledging my feelings to myself. I also began to tell people how important they were to me and to reveal some of my hidden fears. As I did, they began doing the same. With all these efforts, *I began shifting away from seeing myself and my relationships as defined or limited by my physical condition.*

Three specific changes help our relationships with others continue to develop during and after a health challenge:

1. Direct your mind to let go of the idea that someone has to be right and someone has to be wrong.

2. Direct your mind to stop perceiving yourself and people important to you as having separate interests. Instead, direct your mind to perceive that you all have a common goal: to be patient and loving.

3. Be more willing to express yourself and your innermost thoughts and feelings and to listen to others, without fear of abandonment or judgment.

If you commit to seeing *all* interactions as containing opportunities to be more loving (to practice Life-centered thinking), you will transform every interaction into something positive. Though, admittedly, waking up in the morning and not being physically well is not a walk in the park, there is nothing more freeing than waking up each morning knowing that *everything* that is going to happen during the day—regardless if you like it or not—is going to give you the opportunity to be a more centered and loving person.

Asking for Help

In American culture, independence and self-direction are believed to be the highest of all achievements. And during the time following the most difficult aspects of a health challenge, many people tenaciously hang on to this belief. Unfortunately, asking for help of any kind can be seen as a weakness in our society.

Though this problematic idealization of independence holds true across gender lines, it is more firmly established and reinforced in males. Researchers have documented male behavior patterns that arise out of a societal obsession with self-direction, and some of these behaviors border on the ridiculous. For many men, asking for help would be the same as giving up or giving in, either one of which is seen by them as a sign of weakness. If people with this view ask for and accept help during a health challenge, even if they have no choice, their self-esteem will be affected. Interestingly, those who do not ask for help are more likely to suffer longer and not find posttraumatic growth.

Both men and women in American culture have come to live by the tenet "Above all else, be independent." The fact that both men and women in American culture thus lean away from the real need for genuine connection has hardened us and turned us away from Love, the gentle voice of inner wisdom, which often directs us to ask for help. During a health challenge, we need to begin to recognize our interconnectedness with each other and with Love. It is also a time to begin to value the process of asking for help as a way of opening our hearts and the hearts of those we ask.

Asking for help is *not* a sign of weakness or a loss of independence if we keep an open heart. Rather, asking for help taps into the power of friendship, family support, and teamwork. When we consistently turn to Love for support, there are no obstacles we can't overcome during any part of our health challenge.

Directing Your Thoughts and Actions toward Joy

The idea of directing your thoughts and all you do toward joy when you are facing a serious health challenge might sound a bit like asking "Other than that, Mrs. Lincoln, how did you like the play?"

But the truth is, when you blindly choose to follow the ego's way of dealing with a health challenge and put its directives into practice, you will find yourself joyless in about every aspect of your life. Being able to see the end result of the ego's overidentification with the body will help you sort out which thoughts are important for maintaining peace of mind and help you experience joy despite your physical illness. I have seen people in great physical pain, even those preparing to leave this life, be joyful. Consider that moments of joy are possible for you during any phase of your health challenge, and you open a door to a whole different world.

I'm not speaking of the kind of joy that comes from a fun ride at Disneyland or from some pleasurable but temporary experience. I'm speaking of the kind of joy that comes from tapping into the power of Love that is within us, no matter on what ride our life situation is taking us. It is possible for each of us to discover the soft lining of our own hearts, and the hearts of those around us, during the most challenging and painful of times, and it is in this lining that true joy abides. One way to begin tapping into Love is by becoming as aware as possible of the contents of our thoughts and choosing to align our thoughts with Life-centered thinking.

When I was twenty-one, a popular bar offered me a job as an "entrance manager," which was essentially a glorified bouncer.

It was my task to determine at the door who were "appropriate" patrons for the bar and who were not and let in people accordingly. When I made a mistake and let in a troublemaker, it was then my task to tactfully and without incident remove that person from the establishment.

I like to think of my mind as an establishment that is committed to remaining peaceful and coming from Love. I employ a bouncer whose sole purpose is to determine whether or not a certain perception, thought, or belief is conducive to Life-centered thinking. If it is, I gladly let it in. If not, I send it on its way. There is always the chance that the bouncer will make a mistake, and a particularly well-disguised troublemaking thought will get in. In this case, it is necessary for me to tactfully and without incident remove the troublemaking thought from my mind.

During a health challenge, it is particularly important to be able to determine what to let into your mind and what to keep out. Imagine the catastrophe that would occur if medical personnel took no precautions to keep germs out of an operating room. Would you want to go in there? Is it not wise to treat your own mind with the same diligence?

Unfortunately, I have found that the ego also has its own type of bouncer. This bouncer is not really concerned with who or what comes through the door. It is more concerned with keeping our true nature hidden from our awareness. You may well know the bouncer of the ego by another name: *denial.* Its purpose is to build a wall around our mind in order to keep fearful thoughts in and to keep the awareness of Love out. The ego does not want us to see that we are whole and complete, that we are something other than just a body, and that the healing power of Love is available to us at all times, because if we did, the ego would cease to have any power.

But always remember:

The ego and its fear-based thinking may deny the truth of who we are, making us overfocus on our body, but it can't prevent Love from existing everywhere and at all times.

Our willingness to recognize or not recognize certain realities virtually has no effect on their existence. Let's take, for example, the existence of gravity. We cannot *see* gravity. Yet if I denied its existence based on my inability to see this force, the physical reality of gravitational force itself would not in any way be altered. Indeed, it would still influence me.

The force of Life, of Love, is similar to the force of gravity: We may not *see* the force of Life within ourselves, or even experience it because of fear-based thinking, but our inability to see or experience Life does not change the fact that it is everywhere and is always available.

The ego's wishes are meaningless, because the ego's wishes are based on untruths: that fear is real and Love is nowhere. You can pretend that the ego's beliefs are true, but believing does not make it so. Love never abandons you, even if you pretend it has.

While you are facing a health challenge, focus on gaining the willingness and desire to see the truth of who you are and the truth that the force of Life within you is real and is always available. Feel those truths even as you read these words, right now. At this juncture, you needn't concern yourself with whether or not these things are true. You need only decide if you want to believe that they are. You don't have to understand the physics of gravity to experience its effects, nor do you need to fully understand the dynamics of Love to allow it to heal you and bring you peace of mind.

When Pain and Joy Become Confused

The truth is, most people don't really know the difference between what is painful and what is joyful, so they can't consciously choose between the two. Our culture is full of products and actions that promise to bring us joy but ultimately deliver the opposite. When we're first learning to direct our minds, it is very likely we will confuse pain and joy.

Without a doubt, we all would like to believe that we at least know what makes us happy, and we may greatly resist the idea that we don't. I took great offense to the suggestion that, though I was a well-educated person, I did not know what would make me happy. Yet when I learned more, I was surprised at how my real experiences bore out this truth. This "smart guy" spent years choosing pain when the joy of Life was right there, waiting for me.

Discovering my own long history of confusing pain and joy was sobering. From the time I was an adolescent, when I listened to fear-based thinking, I was told that I was incomplete, that I was full of guilt and shame, and that I needed something external to bring me joy. Consequently, I confused pain and joy in three of our culture's most common ways: overusing drugs and alcohol, overidentifying with work, and overidentifying with the body.

All the many ways we confuse pain and joy are the same in that they obscure who we are—Love—and have us look elsewhere for joy, thus causing pain. I spent many years both causing and trying to numb my pain while thinking I was on the path to finding joy. I looked to drugs and alcohol, relationships, work, and the body for joy. Of these, perhaps drugs and alcohol reveal the most when closely examined. Initially, drugs and alcohol seemed to bring me a reprieve from my physical condition and environment, and even the sense of the joy I searched for. In reality, they only took me further away from the true joy of knowing myself through Life-centered thinking. I began to believe, especially because of my health challenge, that the only way I could experience any comfort was if I could get high and escape everything in my life. Not believing joy was possible in any other way, I succumbed to addiction, the ultimate confusion of pain and joy. Eventually, I arrived at a point where I truly felt that either I was going to die or I was going to find something better.

I stopped all the many ways I searched for joy or numbed myself, and when I did, I thought that my pain would cease and joy would rush into my life. What happened was quite the opposite. All the pain I had been hiding from came to the forefront. But this time, I realized that what I had been believing had *caused* my pain. Joy was absent from my life because of what I was believing (i.e., that the only way I could experience any peace of mind was to escape everything in my life), not because of my circumstances. This simple realization provided the foundation for me to begin changing my life, and I have been doing so in the decades since.

What Brings Pain and What Brings Joy

Initially, it may seem as if I'm saying that Life-centered thinking asks you to sacrifice things that are important. It is essential to know that you are asked only to sort out what will bring pain and suffering from what will bring joy and peace of mind. The concern with sacrificing something important to you is part of fear-based thinking. When you become confused about distinguishing what will bring you suffering from what will bring you joy, it may appear to you that Life is just plain inconsistent in bringing you happiness and opportunity. Trust becomes impossible with such an experience.

As mentioned, the ego uses fear to keep us from following the guidance of Life-centered thinking. *Love's guidance becomes equated with fear,* and this connection leads to difficulty in trusting Love, or our inner wisdom, at all. Such is the state of mind I had for years. Having become so fearful and untrusting, a type of emotional and spiritual paralysis set in. It is this paralysis that we must be willing to push through if we are to find true joy.

Truth and Life-centered thinking are perfectly trustworthy. It is only through listening to fear-based thinking that we become confused—to the point that even pain and joy are confused.

Exercise: Sorting Out
What Leads to Pain or Joy

In order to learn to differentiate between pain and joy, begin to practice following a specific assumption or belief to its logical conclusion.

Below is a list of life situations and related assumptions. Even if some of them do not appear to apply to your life, continue with the exercise. Go through them, spending time thinking about the outcome of each one, and then circle *pain* or *joy*. The answers may be rather obvious, but in this period of sorting out what brings pain and what brings joy, it is important to point out the obvious answers to yourself and to constantly remind yourself of their message. This is because you have spent a lot of time doing things and thinking in ways that were obviously not going to lead to joy, just like I did, but we keep doing and thinking in these ways as our denial takes on many different forms.

1. Situation: My _____ (fill in blank with any perceived source of upset, such as your insurance company or a specific person) is being very unreasonable.

Mind-set: I should be defensive and upset about this, and see it/him/her/them as the cause of my upset.

Outcome: Pain / Joy

2. Situation: My spouse/partner is distant today and a bit testy even though I am the one feeling sick.

Mind-set: In my mind, I know that we love each other and are each dealing with my health challenge. I choose to be aware of how much I love my spouse/partner rather than personalize what is happening.

Outcome: Pain / Joy

3. Situation: I am feeling very alone in all this and not supported or understood.

Mind-set: Nobody ever will be there for me, and I should be upset at the world.

Outcome: Pain / Joy

4. Situation: My friends pretty much disappeared when I needed them most, and I was not prepared.

Mind-set: My friends' apparent departure does not reflect how they really feel. I see them as fearful and in need of love and friendship, not judgment and anger.

Outcome: Pain / Joy

5. Situation: I don't feel well, I have to be someplace, and my car won't start this morning. I know that my son used it last.

Mind-set: I should be upset now and for the rest of the day. I should be very angry at my son when I see him. Expressing anger is the best way to vent, feel better, and teach lessons.

Outcome: Pain / Joy

6. Situation: My spouse/partner has a problem, too.

Mind-set: I can help my spouse/partner by listening without judgment or taking on his or her pain.

Outcome: Pain / Joy

7. Situation: I made a mistake in how I have been dealing with my health challenge.

Mind-set: I look at this mistake as an opportunity to learn a lesson. There is no reason to be upset about making a mistake, as getting upset does little good now. Despite my mistake, I know that I am a worthwhile person.

Outcome: Pain / Joy

8. Situation: My doctor did something different from the way I heard another doctor would have done it.

Mind-set: I should tell my doctor what he or she did wrong and that he or she should know another way. And I should get angry, so I can be sure this mistake won't happen again.

Outcome: Pain / Joy

9. Situation: I was taken advantage of during a time I was not feeling well.

Mind-set: I should isolate myself from others and hide in my work. I should always be on the lookout for bad people and should never be vulnerable with anyone.

Outcome: Pain / Joy

10. Situation: My spouse/partner left me after my health challenge became permanent.

Mind-set: I hope he or she feels as bad as I do. I can't trust anyone.

Outcome: Pain / Joy

Again, the outcomes—pain or joy—will likely seem rather obvious to you when the mind-sets are described, because when you look directly at fear-based thinking, it is easy to see how it always leads to pain and suffering. However, ask yourself how many times you have blindly adopted this fear-based thinking in some form, not seeing clearly the inevitable outcome.

It is important to get in the habit of recognizing the pain or joy outcome of *every* thought and belief you have in the same way you recognized their outcomes in this exercise. Even write down your specific thoughts and beliefs and put *pain* or *joy* next to them. Anytime you are upset, sort out your thoughts and beliefs by following the same format in this exercise:

1. State the situation.

2. State the mind-set.

3. State if the mind-set leads to pain or joy.

4. If it leads to pain, write down a mind-set that would lead to joy.

This is a useful exercise to do at the end of each day to practice distinguishing which mind-sets lead to pain and joy so the next day you may choose better. "Sorting out" means being able to look at your own thoughts—daily, if not hourly—the way you sorted the mind-sets in the above exercise. Remember, your skill will improve the more you practice.

Letting Go of Valueless Thinking

If we hold on to what we previously valued (the ego's beliefs), we hinder our ability to learn from new situations, even unwanted ones.

Imagine I wear glasses for nearsightedness, and I get a new prescription because my vision has changed. Upon receiving my new glasses, I still insist on wearing my old ones because I find them to be more comfortable, am used to how I see with them, and believe that they look better. Even though I have what I need to see more clearly, I will not be able to do so until I choose to discard my old glasses, no matter how comfortable they are. It can take a while for us to acclimate to something new, even when it is better for us.

Because most people are both consciously and unconsciously reluctant to give up ways of thinking that they once valued, many try to keep their fear-based way of seeing the world while trying on Life-centered thinking. This is synonymous with putting your new glasses on over your old glasses, and it will not lead to clearer vision.

I remember a scene from *The Jerk,* an old Steve Martin movie, in which he is breaking up with his girlfriend. The setting is the inside of a well-appointed home. He begins by saying, "Well, I'm gonna go then. I don't need any of this! I don't need this stuff! And I don't need you! I don't need anything." On his way across the room to the door, he picks up an ashtray, saying, "Except this. This ashtray. That's the only thing I need." The "except this" routine continues, and by the time he reaches the door, his arms are filled with items, most of which he obviously does not want or need. Though humorous, this scene mirrors how many people approach the step of sorting out their thoughts. We often claim we don't need any fear-based thinking but then hold on to certain schemas even when we know they are not good for us.

Sorting out what is valuable and what is not requires us to work on coming to the present moment, unencumbered by the past. *The most straightforward way we can assess the value of a thought or belief is to determine whether it leads to peace of mind in the present moment.* Relying on the past to determine what is valuable in the present it is like trying to view a fine painting though a dirty glass window.

During even the toughest times of a health challenge, the present moment is the place where our perception can be cleansed by a power greater than ourselves, a place where we can see the value of Life-centered thinking, a sanctuary we can enter to reduce suffering. When we continually have the intention to be in the present moment, over time, the ego becomes like a toothless tiger; its roar becomes little more than a distant whimper.

Because the terms *prayer* and *meditation* can conjure up a variety of ideas, reactions, and definitions, I instead use the phrase "intentional contemplation" to denote two ingredients essential to full healing. We need to utilize the power of *intention* to direct our minds, and we need to use *contemplation* to discover the liberating wisdom that resides within us. Intention is energetically assertive, and contemplation is receptive. The two combined make for a healing force.

The following intentional-contemplation exercise will assist you in continuing to come to the present moment during your health challenge.

Exercise: Intentional Contemplation to Come to the Present Moment

Close your eyes, breathe deeply, and intentionally come with open hands and open heart to the present moment. Say to yourself:

May I listen to the wisdom here, and may it lift me from any suffering, past shame, guilt, or judgment and bring me to see through eyes of Love.

What Is Valuable and What Is Valueless

To help you practice sorting out your thoughts during a health challenge, here are some examples of specific thoughts that are valueless and specific thoughts that are valuable. The following lists are not meant to be complete. Their purpose is merely to aid you in training your mind to more readily recognize what leads to conflict, lack of healing, and fear, and what leads to healing, opportunity, and saying yes to Life.

Remember, *what is valuable leads to peace of mind in the present moment.* Conversely, *what is valueless leads to inner turmoil by promoting overfocus on the body and on the past and future.*

Valueless Thoughts and Beliefs

◆ The more I have, the happier I will be. Obtaining more money, more recognition, more material possessions—this is my goal above all else.

◆ The past is all-important for determining my own self-worth and other people's worth. What someone did in the past is a sure determiner of who she is.

◆ My body must be perfect in order for me to be happy.

◆ Getting old is bad.

◆ We are all separate from one another, with separate interests.

- It is important for me to always succeed, to be better than others, or to have power over the outcome of any situation.

- Other people or circumstances are responsible for how I feel. I am a victim.

Valuable Thoughts and Beliefs

- I have all I need to have peace of mind in this moment. I am complete, and I know there is a power greater than myself.

- In the present moment, I recognize the value of every human being, including myself, regardless of their physical state.

- Health is a state of mind. My happiness primarily depends on my thoughts.

- The essence of who we are, Love, is ageless. Regardless of our age, we all teach one another of Love.

- Material items can disappear over time, but Love, which is everlasting, is unaffected by the passage of time.

- Forgiveness brings me the peace of mind that I want.

- I am responsible for my feelings, my thoughts, and my actions.

In essence, the word *valuable* should only be applied to thoughts and beliefs that are helpful in bringing about understanding, forgiveness, joining, trust, compassion, and Love, all of which bring healing. Valuing the valueless leads to fear, loss, abandonment, isolation, and deep distrust, all of which diminish healing on all levels.

Finding Purpose in All Situations

How much richer our life would be if we always recognized that everything helps us learn the lessons of Love and that nothing is devoid of meaning. Instead, many people go through life continually fighting the things that happen to them, especially if things don't go the way they want. When you're experiencing something you don't particularly want, it is easy to forget that there is potential for growth and learning in every situation.

When I speak to groups of people about this concept, someone in the audience will inevitably come up with examples of situations that they think can't possibly be opportunities for growth and learning. For example, they may say "How about Hitler and the death camps? These can hardly be seen as 'helpful' or 'meaningful.'" Though I certainly agree that horrific, unjust, oppressive situations exist in the world, I am interested in *the response* people are capable of consciously choosing, especially in regard to a health challenge. Though there were people who built and ran the Nazi death camps, there were also prisoners who had the courage and the ability to choose their response, finding meaning even in their catastrophic situation and refusing to be internally or spiritually limited by their circumstance. People throughout history have discovered a deeper faith and commitment to Love in the most catastrophic times. Each of us can become one of these people during our own challenging times.

The work of Dr. Viktor Frankl first opened my eyes to the possibility that the human mind is able to transcend even the worst of atrocities, diseases, and physical hardships. In his writing, Frankl, who survived the terror of the Nazi concentration camps, showed that we are always able to choose how to respond to even the greatest of challenges and to find meaning even in the most painful circumstances.

For me, the idea that we are able to find meaning is of fundamental importance, for it implies a decision to turn inward, to turn to contemplation and compassion, for answers to the deepest questions about what it is to be human. This process of turning inward to find meaning is key during a health challenge.

In one account of his experiences in several concentration camps, including Auschwitz, Frankl said that even under such horribly adverse situations, in which an individual has no control over their circumstances, that person can still determine what will become of themselves both *mentally* and *spiritually*. That means that during our own health challenges, we can always choose to consciously direct our own mind.

In this sense, our destiny and how we live our life do not depend on the external world but rather on *our perception* of that world. In the presence of death and while enduring physical hardships beyond comprehension, Frankl and many others were able to find purpose and meaning in their lives. In his 1959 book *Man's Search for Meaning,* Frankl eloquently and movingly described the power of Love. Observing how he and his fellow prisoners found a reason to live, he wrote:

> *[We saw] the truth—that love is the ultimate and the highest goal to which man can aspire. . . . The salvation of man is through love and in love.*

Frankl went on to describe the way human beings can both create atrocities and transcend them:

> *After all, man is that being who has invented the gas chambers of Auschwitz; however, he is also that being who has entered those gas chambers upright, with the Lord's Prayer or the* Shema Yisrael *on his lips.*

Fear-based thinking would have you believe that unless everything is exactly how *you* think it should be, you cannot be at peace. Fear-based thinking is in a constant battle for control. Nothing else is important to the ego. In contrast, through Life-centered thinking you can begin to see the importance of attitude and intention, through which meaning and purpose can take root and grow in our hearts, thus guiding our lives.

> *There is no situation, no illness, no circumstance that has the power to take away your peace of mind.*

Exercise: Intentional Contemplation to Start Your Day

This intentional contemplation will help you find meaning and purpose in whatever situation you're facing. This contemplation can be a brief and positive way to start your day, even if you are facing large challenges. Try saying it before you even get out of bed.

> *Throughout my day, may I remember that all situations—no matter how they appear or whether or not they are what I wanted to happen—are opportunities to find*

meaning and Love. May I remember throughout this day that there are no circumstances that have any control over my peace of mind, and I choose the thoughts, feelings, and responses I have. If I am challenged, may I choose to turn to my inner wisdom to ask for guidance.

Forgiveness, Compassion, Acceptance: A Life-Centered Philosophy and Practice

Most people have a basic life philosophy that is made up of many unconscious choices, faulty assumptions, and less than accurate feedback from people throughout their life. In sorting out our thoughts during a health challenge, it is important for us to begin thinking about our basic life philosophy, because that philosophy effects how we look at our health challenge. The first part of fully saying yes to Life is to become conscious of our current and past ways of seeing the world and then adopt a Life-centered philosophy.

There are many aspects of the universe that hold much more than meets the eye or even the imagination. In the black holes of the cosmos, time and light play in dimensions that are beyond our usual perception of space and time. Holograms, where two-dimensional images come alive and dance in a three-dimensional space that we can't access, resemble sleight-of-hand magic to the child, yet they are real. Similarly, a Life-centered philosophy is magnificent and very real, and there is much more to it than meets the eye.

I have spent a good deal of my adult life studying and being exposed to people of various cultural backgrounds and spiritual disciplines. Though I do not consider myself to be a scholar in this area, I do feel I have developed the skill of finding common threads running through spiritual traditions and contemporary psychology. For me, sorting out my thoughts has included looking at the commonalities, rather than the differences, between the various paths that lead to significant and peaceful experiences. To some people, the following may seem an oversimplification, but to me, it is a truth that significantly helps me say yes to Life.

I have come to believe that at the base of most any healing path are three interconnected concepts: forgiveness, compassion, and acceptance. These concepts are doorways to understanding trust and finding meaning in life, and they are what have given me the strength to overcome obstacles that once would have stopped me in my tracks. Though I can, and do, speak of the three concepts separately, their true meaning is best experienced when the three are discussed in relation to one another.

At the Base of Most Any Healing Path Are These Three Concepts:

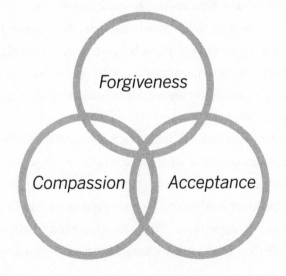

Forgiveness

Within the philosophy of forgiveness is the ability to see when our mind is using comparison as a means of determining self-worth. When dealing with health challenges, many of us fall prey to making constant comparisons: How are we today versus yesterday? How are we compared to how we use to be? How do we compare to other people? What are the statistics? The list can be endless, exhausting, and take us away from the wisdom that is in the quiet of our mind. Comparison implies judgment and usually leads to feelings that originate in fear-based thinking, reinforces low self-worth, and distances us from Life-centered thinking.

The mind that is forgiving strives to see beyond behavior in order to recognize the worth and Love in each individual, including ourselves, at all times, no matter what. This does not mean we have to like someone's behavior or a specific situation or state of being. It simply means that we strive to look within, toward Love. Whereas forgiveness through Life-centered thinking sees a positive future, the ego only sees two possible outcomes: win or lose. With either outcome, it is impossible to consistently have peace of mind because both imply judgment and separation. In terms of dealing with our bodies, having to win increases feelings of unrest, for one day, most all of us must face aging bodies.

In order to sort out our thoughts, it is important to see what forgiveness brings us and what the alternative is. The ego deals in absolutes founded in fear-based thinking. It says, "You are either in good health or bad health," "You are right or wrong," "You are better than or worse than," "You are either liked by everybody or nobody likes you," "You are smart or stupid," "You are good looking or ugly," "You either failed completely or succeeded," "You are either perfect or a complete mess." The list is never ending.

Forgiveness also deals in absolutes, but these absolutes are based in Life-centered thinking. In contrast to the endless list that the ego comes up with, forgiveness always states the same absolute:

Beyond everything that we think did or did not happen, beyond the condition of the body, in each of us is the light of Love.

During a health challenge, our energy is all-important, and pursuing what has no value or what will drain us is, quite literally, a waste of energy. Following a health challenge, many people say something to the effect of "I discovered what was really important to me." I believe what they mean is that all beliefs, reactions, actions, or thoughts that lead them away from having an awareness of the Love within themselves and within other people are valueless.

Compassion

With compassion, the blow with the force of a cannon-ball becomes barely that of a pebble being tossed.

Through the practice of compassion, we recognize and become sensitive to the intimate connectedness of all life. Sometimes when we are most vulnerable, such as during a health challenge, we have the opportunity to experience the deepest compassion for others.

Many people are taught, both directly and indirectly, that force should be met with force and that we should always fight what we don't think should be happening. The problem with this kind of thinking, especially in regard to a health challenge, is that it creates a fearful life in which anger and lack of healing are perpetuated. If we are always fighting or forcing, we become either hardened and tired or shaky, fearful, and without any ability to direct our thoughts toward healing. In dealing with our health, force meeting force is not strength, and total retreat in fear does not create positive change or healing. Both are indications that we do not trust more subtle and gentle ways of responding to the health challenge that has come our way.

Each time we act from something other than compassion—such as from fear, comparison, anger, or resentment—our feelings of being unsafe or ill increase. And, in turn, we build increasingly large defenses. Contrary to the ego's thinking, *defenses always bring that which they were meant to guard against.* Additionally, our defenses distance us from who we are and from our inner wisdom.

To create more options and choices in your life, learn to sort out compassionless thoughts from compassionate thoughts. Once you begin to learn how to respond to all situations with compassion rather than defensiveness, resistance, or force, you are able to redirect your energy toward healing.

I have studied several martial arts throughout the years, and I hold black belts in two. In hakko-ryu and seibukan jujutsu, there is a practice referred to as *henka*. Henka is utilizing your intuition, or *dan*, instead of your intellect to figure out how to respond to whatever situation presents itself. Henka can also be a useful approach to apply when responding to a health challenge. Though the intellect has its place in approaching a health challenge, we should not rely solely on the intellect when responding to a health challenge. The intellect always pauses to assess and analyze the situation. It also tends to respond in rigid, preconditioned, and often fearful ways. Intuition responds in fluid and creative ways because it trusts the Life or Love moving within us. Overthinking and overanalyzing can become dangerous to full healing because they can inhibit this trust.

If we truly allow our intuition and inner wisdom to respond to our health challenge, there will be no compassionless thinking in our lives. In contrast, to the degree that we do not trust our intuition—the power of our inner wisdom—will be the degree to which we will not have full healing and will remain in fear.

Compassionless thinking creates a lack of trust in our inner wisdom. At a certain point in my own healing journey, I was forced to see the effects of compassionless thinking. I wanted to sort out the resentful feelings I held about other people and my feelings about myself, because I saw how these feelings held me back in all areas of my life and interfered with healing. The problem was that I wasn't feeling anything. I could talk endlessly *about* things, but I greatly resisted feeling anything. I think somewhere along the line I had decided to put up an "out of business" sign on my feelings.

Then one day, largely due to the vulnerability that came from struggling with my illness, I began to cry. The sounds that left my body were ones I had never heard before. They came from deep within, from the center of my being. Sounds of pain filled the room, my whole universe. Time changed dimensions. I could have been there for an hour or a minute; I didn't know. All my hidden pain, which had caused me to be angry and resentful, began to pour out with those sounds. Tears finally found their way out of me in a genuine way.

Based on this experience, I developed an intentional contemplation that I find very helpful. This intentional contemplation, through taking Love in, allows us to release suffering and replace it with compassion for the world. It is quite simple, but its results are profound.

Exercise: Intentional Contemplation for Releasing Suffering

Sit and focus on your breath. On the inhale say "I breathe in Love." On the exhale say "I breathe out suffering." After several minutes, as you settle into this rhythm, say "I breathe in Love," and on the exhale say "I give compassion to all."

As long as I was afraid of my pain, I kept it hidden. My pain had previously weighed me down in everything I did, and eventually it bred one compassionless thought after another. My hidden pain and suffering turned to blame and feelings of powerlessness. In my day-to-day activities, I was unaware of the energy I expended in order to keep my suffering and fear repressed, but it became clear that my life was void of vitality and healing because of it. Moving through my fear of what was inside of me opened up choices. This process *always* leads to compassionate thinking. Remember the following two facts:

1. When you bring suffering and fear to the calmness of your inner wisdom, you transform them into compassion for yourself and others. This compassion leads to healing.

2. When you keep your suffering (such as anger, guilt, and resentments) hidden, it breeds compassionless thinking that keeps you stuck and unable to bring about full healing.

Acceptance

With the practice of acceptance, we find a place within ourselves that prepares us for letting go, which is part of the healing process. The philosophy of acceptance is the heart of a spiritual path, as reflected in part of the Serenity Prayer, "Grant me the serenity to accept the things I cannot change, courage to change the things I can, and wisdom to know the difference." Further, acceptance is seeing the light of Love in someone, regardless of the circumstances.

Acceptance, like forgiveness, is *not* a passive position in which we accept negative situations that can be improved or behavior that is damaging. Rather, it is an *active* position wherein we identify with the truth of who we are and empower ourselves to focus our energy on creating the peace of mind we want. Thus, acceptance allows us to

- overcome unnecessary confrontation;
- see kindness and strength as connected;
- release the victim role;
- become humble;
- never attack, never defend, and take care of ourselves while seeing the worth of others;
- know that strength comes from respecting ourselves and others, knowing ourselves, being light on the planet, and

having the courage to bring positive change to our lives and the world.

Our basic survival as humans depends on our individually and collectively adopting an attitude of acceptance—of seeing Life in all things. If we don't, increasingly violent wars and environmental problems will be givens. Unfortunately, the current global environmental crisis and level of international conflict show that we have taken another, more precarious path. We tend to treat our own bodies and minds poorly, and we are similarly ravaging the Earth and depleting its resources. In the same way that many people pollute their beings with fearful thinking and their bodies with junk food and sedentary lifestyles, we injure the very air that we breathe and clear-cut forests, yet blind ourselves to the ill effects of our actions. When we fully embrace healing for ourselves, we will also embrace healing for the planet.

Adhering to the philosophy of acceptance reveals an important path—one where understanding that cutting down an acre of rain forest in Brazil affects the entire planet or that holding on to one fear-based thought affects every part of our health and those around us. To accept Love is to accept the power of a solution and of being kind and gentle in all ways and to become aware that everything on Earth is intimately connected. Coming to this realization is a key part of the healing journey that is saying yes to Life.

Causing harm—which is to say, perpetuating fear—can be seen as the opposite of acceptance. Harming ourselves or other human beings in the ways described above is a primary obstacle to healing. Our ego tells us that getting what we think we want is what is important, but it doesn't tell us that it has no real idea what is good for us. How else could we so blindly pollute our minds, bodies, and the planet? Upon closer examination, it is obvious that this behavior never gives us lasting peace of mind; by always perpetuating fear, it limits health and healing. Accepting the true nature of someone or ourselves—Love—beyond behavior or physical circumstances is what heals. Without the gentleness and compassion that come with the adoption of acceptance, not only will our healing be limited, but also our species may not survive.

Our healing is, in part, based on changing our mind and our thoughts to be more in line with the philosophy of acceptance. Admittedly, this change is not always easy in our culture. Our world has become so used to thinking that controlling, overpowering, fighting, and forcing bring us safety that we apply this same approach to health care, which can impede rather than foster full healing. When it comes to our health, often the primary concern is with aggressive physical interventions. This is not to say that aggressive medical treatment has no place, but simply that it alone cannot bring us full healing, life transformation, and learning.

Fear-based thinking seeks false strength or healing through domination, attack, and control. The philosophy of Life-centered healing promotes full healing through acceptance, compassion, and forgiveness, as well as the gentleness and kindness they produce.

CHAPTER NINE

Step Two: Letting Go

Letting Go of What Holds Us Back from Health

Even when we're ready to find a better way and say yes to Life, there is still a part of us that firmly believes fear-based thinking is our only road to surviving a health challenge, and this belief gets in the way of our healing. This chapter is concerned with letting go of what no longer serves us.

To illustrate the importance of this step, consider the following example. Under my kitchen sink, I have containers into which I sort garbage from what can be recycled. This effort is worthwhile, though incomplete in itself. It is incomplete because if I never took out the garbage or visited the recycling center, all my sorting out would result only in a very stinky kitchen.

The same is true with our thinking. If we sort out our thoughts into which are fear-based and which are Life-centered but never let go of the fear-based thinking, our minds will not be all that different from my stinky kitchen.

Because most people tend to be fairly set in their ways of thinking and behaving, and because during stress, such as the stress that comes with a health challenge, we tend to revert to old patterns, it is rare that we let go of our old beliefs, reactions, and assumptions without a certain amount of despair. For this reason, letting go takes courage. It also calls on and reinforces our commitment to peace of mind.

Letting Go Is the Threshold to Healing

Perhaps the greatest suffering during a severe health challenge comes from the inability to let go of the desire to control all aspects of our experience.

In modern times, most people grow up learning a set of values that directly oppose the principle of letting go of what inhibits trust in our life and healing. We are often taught that accumulating, acquiring, achieving, holding on, getting more, and keeping what we have are the hallmarks of success. We come to believe that learning is a process of filling our minds with information until no more will fit, then packing just a little more in, and then performing on some outside measure, such as a test, that is unintentionally given far more weight than the learning itself. Kids hardly have time to be kids anymore. By middle school, they are feeling undue pressure and worrying about a future that seems uncertain rather than learning the value of experiencing grace in the moment, being supported in positively stretching their comfort zones without fear of negative consequences, and learning to value the internal experience of service above external validation. From an early age, we are taught that past performance and mistakes are very important and that being concerned about the future to the point of excessive worry is an act of being responsible. The problem with this kind of education is that there is little or no emphasis on living in the present moment or developing grace, compassion, and trust in our inner wisdom. In other words, when we are faced with a health challenge, we are not prepared for healing.

True healing—be it on a personal, interpersonal, or a global level—is, in part, a process of sorting out and letting go. This is a difficult process because fear-based thinking tells us that we're nuts if we turn away from its platform. *In order to have health and healing, we must be willing to let go of what we have deemed valueless.*

There is no point in sorting out the valuable from the valueless if we don't take the next logical step. Letting go is the threshold of peace of mind. In this respect, forgiveness and letting go are similar.

If we view letting go as *giving up what we think will make us happy,* it will generate conflict. Sometimes a toddler cries when a toy is taken away, even if that "toy" happened to be something dangerous. In this same way, during a health challenge, we adults can become quite upset when we think that we are giving up some thought, belief, way of acting, physical ability, or possession that we believe we cannot be happy without, even though it may be very harmful and inhibit healing.

Letting go does not mean becoming passive, nor does it mean developing an attitude of disengagement. Letting go does, however, require something that is very different and difficult for most people: It requires releasing our belief that something has to be a certain way for us to have peace of mind. Such thoughts, and the actions that stem from them, take us on a wild goose chase. Deciding to focus on what *can* improve our health—*our responses* to our situation—is the only way to empowerment and to Life-centered living.

The Life-centered responses we develop as we let go of our fear-based thoughts and need to control are based on what humanistic psychologist Carl Rogers termed *unconditional positive regard.* This means looking beyond what we believe is bad, beyond illness, or beyond negative self-image and toward the Love that shines within us all, however obscured it may be. A central part of Life-centered living is choosing to let go of all the thinking that relentlessly condemns us for what we have done in the past. In other words, we need to let go of our self-imposed guilt if we wish to truly say yes to Life.

Fear's Favorite Trick

I have always loved magic and over the years have learned a few magic tricks. I realized early on that most illusions have one thing in common: They redirect the audience's attention so that the audience will not see what the magician is actually doing.

The ego and fear-based thinking play tricks on our mind each and every day, especially during a health challenge. They redirect our attention so we will not see that the decision to suffer is merely a smoke-and-mirrors act. The favorite trick of the ego and fear-based thinking is to convince us the source of pain is where it is not. The real source of inner pain is the belief that we are separate from Love, but the ego and fear-based thinking always direct our attention to an illusion or a problem of some sort.

The ego's four big tricks are shame, anger, the body, and guilt. They are presented in a way that makes them appear to be very real, all-consuming, and insurmountable. The master dark magician, the ego, finds ways to divert our attention from the true source of our pain—our thinking—and away from healing. Magicians call such diversion redirection; psychologists call it displacement; Eastern spiritual traditions call it *maya*. Whatever the act of diversion is called, the point of it is to keep us believing in the illusion.

The ego's grandest illusion during a health challenge is that we are our bodies. This mother of all illusions comes in a variety of forms. Recently I was speaking with a woman named Alison, who continued to feel that she was not and would never be happy because of a double mastectomy. She told me how since the removal of her breasts, she could not think of much else besides her scarred body. Though a period of grieving is needed after such a procedure, hers had gone on for a very long time, and she still felt depressed and stuck two years later. What she did not see was how her thinking was just a manifestation of her ego's favorite illusion—the idea that she was her body and that she was not okay how she was *right now*.

In order to begin to let go of this illusion—and, thus, to heal—she needed to first clearly see the problem and the solution.

The problem is always the same: The ego, through fear-based thinking, uses a belief that you are your body and the illusions of guilt and shame to keep you from seeing all of who you are.

The solution is always the same: Know you are Love. Know you have a body, but you are much more than your body. Know that you have a past, but you are not defined by your past.

One aspect of healing for Alison was for her to be able to say "I am a woman who has great passion but has been lured away from it by overfocusing on my body defining who I am. I will now take the time to find out who I am." Alison is learning that letting go of the illusions of fear-based thinking allows her to become increasingly present in the moment, without judgment and condemnation. Being present in the moment clears the path for Love, healing, and a self-image that is based on more than just her body.

Kids love magic, but if they figure out the trick, they are quick to tell you. I suggest that when we see the ego doing one of its tricks, no matter how large the illusion is, we respond as kids do: "Come on, not *this* trick again." Once we see the illusion, the trick no longer has power, and we can let go of anything other than the truth.

Recognizing the ego's illusions is a big part of letting go, and letting go becomes much easier as we practice it. Think of it this way: When you ask the ego a question about health and healing, it is liking asking a stranger for directions and getting pointed in the opposite direction of where you want to go. The ego points us everywhere but to the thoughts that we need to let go. In contrast, Life-centered thinking always points us in the right direction—toward trusting our inner wisdom and who we really are.

Healing as a Time of Letting Go of Guilt

During a health challenge, it is easy for us to feel guilty for many things or to make other people feel guilty. Earlier in my life, during a health challenge, I was a master at making the other person in a relationship feel guilty. I irrationally and unconsciously believed that making another person feel guilty would lessen my load. In other words, I displaced the guilt I was feeling about being sick and the effects my illness was having on my family onto someone else, thinking that this displacement would make me feel better.

I did the same thing with anger. I would actually invent things to be angry about, though I would seldom admit to myself or to the other person that I was doing so. Without thinking about it,

I would be on the lookout for situations in which I could become angry. It was as if I had a pressure cooker of anger inside of me because of my health, and I had to find some "justifiable" way to let off some of the steam.

One such event took place many years ago, but I remember it well because it represents so well how little I was following Life-centered thinking. I was dating a woman whom I was very serious about. We had plans that involved spending our lives together, and my health challenge was interrupting them. I felt that I was doing everything right in my life and it was not fair that I had become ill. As my partner grew increasingly distant from me, she assured me that she was simply going through a lot inside in response to my health and that everything would work out if I would be patient.

I believed that my anger was justified, that I was the one sick, and that everybody would surely agree with me. Armed with self-righteousness, I became furious about the situation. I felt I was being abandoned, and I confronted my partner about it. I was verbally abusive to her, and my single goal was to make her feel guilty and wrong. I wanted to punish her.

The result was that we both felt a lot of things, but neither of us experienced any peace of mind. In letting go, it is important to realize that even the most justifiable anger does not result in peace. Eventually that relationship ended. It was not until years later, after many more episodes of self-righteous anger directed at other people, that I began to look for the deeper source of my anger—guilt, shame, and helplessness. It would be even more years before I turned to Love to help me forgive myself and other people and to help me see that the state of my body had nothing to do with the state of my mind.

I have learned that guilt and shame, no matter how intense they seem, are nothing more than illusions. Through experience, I have also learned that anytime I try to project my guilt on another person, the result will be increasing my own guilt and inner conflict. The truth is:

If I see guilt in any relationship, including my relationship with myself, it is because I have put it there.

Guilt is poison to any relationship.

During a health challenge, many relationships suffer greatly. If during your recovery from a health challenge you do not examine your anger, guilt, and shame, you will continue to believe in the illusion that they are real and that Love is not ever present within you. And if you do not let go of this belief, you will inevitably displace your guilt and shame, seeing others as guilty and unworthy of your understanding and compassion. The main purpose of displacement is to convince you that the source of your guilt is outside of yourself and beyond your control. How can you let go of that which lies beyond your grasp?

Displacement is the ego's idea of letting go. But it actually chains us to guilt, and guilt chains us to the past. With guilt, we cannot completely know Love, and we cannot recognize Love in others nor share forgiveness, compassion, and acceptance. In other words:

When we believe in guilt and fear, we will not believe in letting go of them or seeing the power of Love. Happiness and healing will thus escape us.

Exercise: Intentional Contemplation for Committing to Letting Go of Guilt and Shame

I invite you to make the following commitment:

I, regardless of my physical or mental condition, will no longer use any relationship to hold myself to the past by valuing guilt. I will not try to punish others by attempting to make them feel guilty, nor will I try to punish myself in this manner. I will not use shame as an irrational reason to not look within or to attack another person. I make the commitment to let go of guilt and shame because I believe that letting them go is the foundation for healing and a healthy life.

"If My Eyes Looked through Love, What Would I See?"

Asking this question takes us beyond the condition of our body and expresses a commitment to giving new, healthy vision a priority in our lives.

In order to see things through Love's eyes, we must let go of our old way of seeing. Many people who are in the midst of a health challenge live in a conflicted state of mind much of the time, and the thought of Love does not occur to them on a regular basis, if ever. Despite the discomfort this state of mind brings, we may feel reluctant to practice Life-centered thinking because we are still attached to the way that we see things, even though that way is not working well for us.

At this stage of letting go of our old fear-based thinking, the purpose is simply to bring the awareness of Love a little closer than it was yesterday. If you find yourself tempted to think that this idea asks you to give up something desirable, contemplate this:

If my eyes were the eyes of Love, what would I see?

Love has no cost to anyone.

It will lead to only increased trust, peace, and compassion.

I suggest that you write down these words, carry them with you, and repeat them to yourself many times throughout the day, especially when you are upset about your health challenge and physical condition. Remember that simply asking yourself this question, "If my eyes looked through Love, what would I see?" especially in difficult situations, will help you to find a new way—Love's way—of viewing yourself and the world.

Do not be hard on yourself if you find yourself forgetting to ask this question and becoming entangled in your thoughts about your physical health. Rather, thank yourself for reintroducing the idea and then try to keep the focus. At this point, if you ask sincerely, just one time, to see through Love's eyes, you will be opening the door to a whole new outcome for your current situation.

Developing the willingness to see anything, including your body and anyone your eyes rest on, in a different way whenever you are not at peace—the way Love would have you perceive it—will serve you well. Asking to see all the events in your day through Love's eyes—or, for that matter, to see even one small event differently—is a useful exercise for opening your mind to the present moment and to the power of Love, unencumbered by fear and worry.

When we ask to see something through Love's eyes, we commit to ceasing to define ourselves by the state of our bodies or by what has occurred in the past. When we turn within and ask to see an experience from Love's perspective, instead of continuing to see it through the lens of our past experiences, assumptions, and expectations, we will create a distinctly different experience.

Creative problem-solving is often referred to as thinking outside the box. Creativity and bona fide problem-solving, really thinking outside the box, are directly related to asking our inner wisdom for a different perception than the one we had when we were experiencing suffering. For example, if I bind the meaning of something as simple as a chair to my limited experience of chairs, I will probably miss many creative opportunities that someone else may see. The artist may notice a chair's unique form. The woodworker may become fascinated by the subtle patterns of the chair's wood grain. The child may become excited by the idea of using the chair to make a jungle gym or a fort.

Thinking outside the box is a direct result of letting go of our preconceived ideas about something, someone, or a situation. Once we do, the creative force within us comes forth. In my experience, this creative force comes from something much larger than ourselves. Thinking outside the box by asking to see through Love's eyes is incredibly useful when approaching a health challenge, because it can help us find a unique purpose in each day and even within the health challenge itself.

Asking to see through Love's eyes is important to healing of any kind. Many times we assume we know all about a situation or person instead of seeing it, him, or her in light of the present moment. *The greatest mistake we can ever make is thinking that because we have certain thoughts and reactions about our health challenge, we know all of what should or should not happen.*

Just as an astronomer would never look through a telescope and say "I know all about the universe and all that lies beyond it," we must never look at another human being or our health challenge and think that we fully know the depth of who that person is or all the details of the situation. Instead, we must let go of what we think we know, turn to Love, and simply ask for clearer vision.

Letting Go of Health-Blocker Thoughts

As you recall, fear-based thoughts can be considered as blocks to healing and health—as health-blocker thoughts. The good news is that, like ice set in the direct sun, health-blocker thoughts melt to nothing and evaporate if we are willing to bring them into the light of Love. With the letting go of fear, Love is free to be present in our lives, and that is the basis for health.

We need to measure our progress not by how close we come to never having any negative thoughts in response to our health challenge, but by how willing we are to recognize what we are doing and by how willing we are to let it go and choose a Love-based perception of the situation. Anytime you are not experiencing peace of mind, go through the following three steps:

1. **Ask yourself, "What health-blocker thoughts (such as shame, guilt, resentment, revenge, worry, or feelings of inadequacy) am I having right now?"**

Examples: "The doctor is completely inconsiderate for being late, and I have every right to be angry." "I am a failure for not having prepared financially for something like this." "I can't possibly be happy after this kind of surgery." "If tomorrow's test does not go well, all will be ruined."

2. **Tell yourself, "These thoughts are untrue, are not helping me, and are blocking healing."**

Picture a giant stop sign in your mind, illustrating that you want to stop this thinking. If you really want to use your imagination, picture a couple of angels holding up the stop sign for you to see, or picture yourself placing your health-blocker thoughts into a celestial garbage bin. Alternatively, you can do what a dear friend of mine does: She pictures a grocery store with aisles marked with signs saying, "Worries," "Judgments," and "Anger." If she realizes that somehow she has accumulated a basket full of such thoughts, she returns them to the proper aisles and commits to not picking them up again. She is then free to go to the aisles marked "Forgiveness," "Compassion," and "Understanding" and fill her basket to the brim.

3. **Ask your inner wisdom for a different way of seeing the situation that is concerning you.**

Examples: "The doctor's tardiness gives me an opportunity to spend a much-needed moment with myself." "Love is shining in me now, and the condition of my body does not reflect my worth." "I can let go of all self-imposed limitations if I am willing."

Practicing the following two intentional contemplation exercises will further set your mind in the direction of healing.

Exercise: Intentional Contemplation for Letting Go

During this challenging time, may I look gently on myself and others. May faith in Love help me find meaning in my health challenge, regardless of the condition of my body. May I listen to my inner wisdom, not the chatter of my fear, anger, and guilt. May I not be deceived or bound by my ego and fearful thinking insisting that I should be very upset. May I know deep in my soul that through letting go, I will discover the quiet and peaceful path that is now open to me, and I will follow it willingly.

Exercise: Intentional Contemplation for the Courage to Live a Life of Purpose

During this challenging time, may I have the wisdom to release my own and other peoples' expectations and fears so that I can find what it is true for me. May I have the courage to choose to see the lessons my life brings rather than living a life of doing only what other people think I should do.

CHAPTER TEN

Step Three: Settling Down

It's as if we've been at sea in a severe winter storm, in a boat that has lost its rudder. Finally the sun breaks through, the waves die down, and land is spotted.

When we commit ourselves to saying yes to Life, including consistently practicing sorting out and letting go, we eventually begin to feel the positive effects of our efforts. When we navigate through our health challenges with increasing kindness, faith, and trust in Love, an uncommon sense of calm comes to us. It is important to value this, above almost all other things in our lives, or it can easily be lost again.

Value Stillness within Yourself

As I've traveled and spoken to many large groups of people, I have seen numerous courageous souls who are very committed to their healing. Though this commitment to healing is a good thing, during a health challenge we can become so used to working on healing, personal growth, and taking care of the details of life that we sometimes end up thinking that if we are not struggling with these issues, something is wrong. It is not uncommon to become suspicious of any stillness or calm in our lives, like parents get nervous when the kids are too quiet.

It is also common to find that when our health challenge begins to settle down, we don't know what to do with our time anymore, having spent so much of it on treatments, doctor visits, discussions, and so on. Many people mistakenly think they need to have some drama to focus on in their lives. Struggling with a long-term health challenge begins to feels normal, and when it is gone, there is a void.

Some individuals have been waiting for the day they finally find all the answers. They dislike any kind of internal struggle. When they at last feel the struggle subside, they are convinced that they have completed their inner journey and arrived at some magical destination where conflict and old patterns will never again affect them. The eventual letdown, which is often major, comes when they find that their peace of mind has not yet been fully established. These people become quite disillusioned when the next thing in life, often a continuation of the health challenge, again unsettles them.

The important thing to remember is when a health challenge begins to move to the next phase (no matter what direction the challenge takes), there is a time of consolidation. It is a time to implement what we have learned thus far, apply it to our lives to the best of our ability, and then continue to move forward. Curiously, this time of consolidation happens regardless of what physical changes there might be. For example, those who are returning to work need a time of consolidation, as do those who are preparing for death.

Become Present-Based to Have Health Memories

During childhood, many people learn that conditional love is the only love that exists. Parents can sometimes unwittingly teach children that love is tied to performance rather than being.

Performance-based child-rearing, which is the opposite of Life-centered parenting, teaches that if children meet certain expectations, they will be deserving of love. The children hear the covert message that being loved depends on their satisfying another person's expectations and desires. In adulthood, a performance-based approach to our identity leads only to fear and an endless pursuit of acceptance and approval from others. To varying degrees, these dynamics play out during a health challenge; we can feel less than whole and lovable when we are dealing with all that ill health can bring.

Conversely, Life-centered child-rearing teaches children that Love lives in them in this present moment, and that there is no child or adult who does not deserve to be loved. One mark of being on a true healing path as adults is seeing that our self-worth is not dependent on accomplishments or achieving some specific look or state of physical health. It is never too late to recognize that Love is within us, and it is precisely this recognition that leads to true healing.

Also important is the realization that performance-based approaches to health all have to do with getting some physical result, and often we are very attached to having that result, believing that without it, happiness would be impossible.

For the development of health, it is imperative that we understand the difference between performance-based and Life-centered approaches to healing.

If we don't understand this difference and its application to our health challenge, we only continue to view health as some kind of reward we get or don't get because of something we do or don't do. In a performance-based approach to health, the ego sets us on this reward-seeking journey, which will eventually lead to hopelessness and despair.

Some of this discussion can be easily misunderstood, because in our culture there is so much emphasis on medical intervention and modern technology. It should be noted that the benefits that come from modern medicine are good things. I personally would not be here without them. *Performance-based approaches only become problematic when we equate our self-worth and self-esteem to how well our physical body is healing or its current state.*

Insane results come from insane thinking, and in this case, we will seek but never find the happiness and health we are craving. This endless cycle is certainly not joyous, and it is most certainly not conducive to finding health as defined as inner peace. In a Life-centered approach to health, the roots of true healing are seeing ourselves as more than just our bodies, in the light of the present moment.

Up until now, you may have been following the irrational "seek but do not find" health plan of the ego because you knew no other way, not to mention because it appears to be a very popular plan in our culture. You may not remember how to look within and to Love for healing, for the simple reason that you don't believe your source of health is there. Yet there is a part of you that does remember, and that part will faithfully guide you toward true health. Most often the word *memory* denotes the image of something that happened in the past. But the memory of how to look within and to Love for healing is a "health memory," one that is beyond linear time and that can be remembered in different ways, including through a health challenge.

All that we need to trigger this health memory is a willingness to turn away from the ego and toward Love, which awaits us in the everlasting present moment. It is only our mind that believes in the ego and gives reality to it and its fear-based health-blocker thoughts. Yet it is also our mind that can choose to turn away from the ego and toward Love. Our health challenge, despite all its difficulties, can be a time of settling down with Love, when much of our attention is focused on remembering who we are.

For many years, I had no idea that I was something more than my body and that there was something more than the physical world: I had a spiritual home that Love kept safe for me as it awaited my return. Or if I did, that home was just an abstract concept. For much of my life, I believed there was an emotional price to pay for love. I believed either I had to do something or sacrifice something in order to be loved. I spent much of my time chasing after accomplishments, trying to be "healthy," or denying a part of myself, including my health challenge, in order to be accepted. In short, I did not feel lovable, and I certainly did not feel happy. I was secretly convinced that if I was not producing or achieving through work, or if I became more ill, Love would be withdrawn.

Slowly and gratefully, I have learned that I was mistaken. I have come to know that Love is neither earned nor withheld; it is simply to be recognized and accepted, or not. I have found that deciding who I am at this moment, no matter what my physical circumstance, is the most important decision I can make. If I decide I am defined by the past or my body, I will not trust myself, and I will not turn to my inner wisdom, Love.

Recognizing and accepting Love is something we decide to do every minute of every day. And whether or not we do always depends on our belief about who we are.

Love is the source of healing.

How to Find Quiet in Chaos

The period of facing a health challenge is not typically a quiet time but rather is full of important decisions and overwhelming emotions. Yet quiet is exactly what is needed during much of this time.

One of the main problems we encounter when beginning to pursue Life-centered thinking is that we are simply unaccustomed to having a calm and quiet mind. We may actually be a bit uncomfortable with tranquility, feeling that we *should* be doing something at all times. We don't trust the quiet. We may even be bored, because we are limited in our physical and daily activities. We may have become so used to a busy mind that anything else seems abnormal. But until we recognize that we are avoiding quiet, we will find problems to be solved, drama to involve ourselves in, resentments to build, worry to consume us, and self-condemnation to collect, none of which serves your health and healing.

When dealing with a health challenge, we need to treat our tranquility as though it were a beautiful estate for which we are the caretakers. Anytime weeds or unwanted intrusions present themselves, we must be quick to deal with them in order to maintain our tranquility.

Although being with other people is important, it is also important that we spend time alone. Indeed, with the busy schedules that can accompany a health challenge, many people spend very little time alone. And even when they do, they are often task oriented, spending their solitude doing such things as reading or learning about their condition.

In our society today, we have books, movies, the Internet, and endless other entertainment options. We are often quick to fill our free time with some form of task or amusement. During a health challenge, when it is easy to either be busy dealing with the logistics or to zone out with entertainment of some kind, we need to recognize the real reason we might constantly need to be entertained and/or distracted: to be taken away from ourselves. It may be that we have become fearful of being alone and uncomfortable without distractions. This is the way of the ego: It convinces us that we should be afraid of what is inside of us—of Love, of Life, of our inner wisdom—in order to keep us searching outside ourselves.

Though many free-time choices are certainly helpful (because they are creative expressions), they can also distract us from saying yes to Life. You may have heard financial planners suggest, "Take at least 10 percent of your income and set it aside for savings and investments. Do this no matter what is going on financially, and when you sit down to pay your bills, always pay yourself first. If you do this, along with deciding to live more simply, financial freedom will come." While there is much more to financial investing, without this basic approach, the goal of financial freedom is hard to achieve. The same ingredients of this straightforward financial advice apply to saying yes to Life.

Exercise: Invest 5 Percent of Your Time in Settling Down with Love

Take at least 5 percent of your waking hours—more on some days—and set it aside for being alone, settling down, and turning within, *without any task to do or entertainment to distract you.* Your sole purpose during this time is to settle down with Love. Do this no matter how chaotic your life is, how much you have to do, how bad you feel, or how behind you think you are. When you schedule your day, always set time aside for yourself first. Though there is much more to your healing path and to saying yes to Life, making this simple commitment will enable you to find much more quiet and calm in the midst of chaos. Just as you need a charged battery on a cell phone to pick up signals and transmissions, you need a receptive and quiet mind to hear the guidance of Love that is always available to you. Although Love is with us at all times and in all places, we typically need to have a quiet mind to receive it.

To develop trust in Love, commit to spending time—contemplative time—without distractions. Be willing to begin to spend time settling down with Love. The ego is very skilled at creating both external and internal distractions. Make the 5 percent commitment, and your life will be 95 percent improved. Now that's the best investment deal going.

When my daughters were small, they used to be enraptured with the magic of snow globes. When the snow globe was shaken, the scene inside would turn to a snowy wonderland; flecks of white would fall over the town inside the liquid world. They would watch with fascination as the snow slowly settled, and then, just before stillness, they would shake it up again, laughing and giggling.

Our ego and fear-based thinking do something similar. They are always shaking up our minds, for no other reason than that stillness is as dangerous to the ego as water is to fire. If you get close to stillness, the ego will surely find a way to entice you to shake things up.

Love comes to us in the stillness of our mind. The ego knows this and is threatened by it, so it is always throwing distraction in our way. With a health challenge, the ego appears to have an endless supply of material to use to shake up our minds. The moment we may begin to feel some stillness, the ego will try and pull our attention to some physical concern, pain, or worry.

Lead Feelings

In our health-care culture, people facing a health challenge are met with a blitz of distractions. But our health-care culture provides very little, if any, time and support for people wanting to find and explore their inner life or develop a Life-centered focus. As a result, people are living longer but are less happy, and many are "lost souls" as they transition from this life.

I know what this lost, unhappy state is like because I was one of these people. There were times during my early health challenges when trying to feel something other than depression, numbness, anger, or resentment would have been nearly impossible.

It is difficult to experience healing when we are full of fear and have no trust in Love, and our minds are full of worry and dread.

During the process of settling down, we begin to be more aware of all aspects of ourselves and our lives, even though our health challenge remains a central focus. In particular, our feelings become more available to us, because we do not have the thoughts and distractions that previously kept us from experiencing them.

In many personal-growth experiences, a great emphasis is put on what the individual is feeling. I agree with this emphasis in part. Yet so often, as was the case with me, when we are asked, "What are you feeling?" the question might as well be "What does the other side of Mars look like?" Many people are so out of touch with their feelings, especially in the midst of facing a health challenge, that they don't even know where to start or why they should bother exploring their feelings.

The reason we bother is because feelings and beliefs are very closely related. It is important to see how what I call *lead feelings* and *core beliefs* can create a life of happiness and healing or a life of suffering and illness.

A lead feeling is a feeling that results from a specific belief. Our ego tells us that certain feelings, such as shame and fear, are not just feelings, but *who we are*. During those years I experienced a lot of shame, it did not feel like a transitory feeling. I believed that *who I was* was shameful. With a belief such as this, who would want to experience any more feelings? When shame is at the core of who we believe we are, any experience of any feeling only increases our sense of shame. By adulthood,

I had become so guarded and distant that I was rarely able to access what I was feeling at any specific time, especially when I first faced a physical challenge.

Core beliefs cause lead feelings, and then the lead feelings reinforce the original core beliefs. They strengthen each other. Together, they affect all other facets of our lives, including our inner lives.

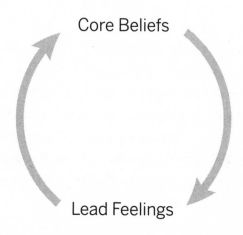

Fortunately, like thoughts, lead feelings can also be positive and health-centered. Love is the primary Life-centered lead feeling. Stemming from Love, then, are the positive experiences and expressions of compassion, joy, and peace.

Exercise: Intentional Contemplation for Creating Life-Centered Lead Feelings

Because our core beliefs determine our lead feelings, it is extremely important to address our beliefs. I suggest beginning each day by reading the following intentional contemplation.

Today may I settle down with the awareness of Love
through feeling compassion for myself and others,
kindness in my heart,
genuine gentleness within my soul,
and deep gratitude for my life,
no matter the condition of my body.

◇

Below are some more examples of core beliefs that produce lead feelings of shame, fear, and guilt, and then examples of core beliefs that produce Life-centered lead feelings. A good rule of thumb: Any thought that creates separation is fear-based; any thought that creates joining is Life-centered. When we experience Life-centered feelings, our fear-based feelings dissipate, creating emotions of safety that allow us to settle down with Love.

True health is not fearing any aspect of ourselves.

Negative Core Beliefs That Produce Lead Feelings of Shame, Fear, or Guilt (Suffering)

1. During a health challenge, it is better to be quiet and always make sure that everybody is happy.

2. During a health challenge, I should never show emotion, because doing so is a sign of weakness.

3. During a health challenge, I should never make waves but always be agreeable and a peacekeeper.

4. Negative experiences can never be overcome.

5. If I begin to focus on feelings during a health challenge, I will be overcome with negative feelings.

6. Other people are responsible for how I feel.

7. My body is not how I want it to be, and it is shameful.

8. During a health challenge, trying anything new or different will lead to failure.

9. What I feel is wrong. Expressing my feelings is not a good idea.

10. I am not worthy of love.

Positive Core Beliefs That Produce Lead Feelings of Compassion, Kindness, and Gratitude (Release from Suffering)

1. During a health challenge, it is okay for me to have a voice. Everybody does not need to approve of my choices for me to feel good about myself.

2. During a health challenge, forgiveness is a strong position.

3. During a health challenge, disagreements do not indicate anything about me or the other person. My goals are always understanding and joining, even in disagreements.

4. During a health challenge, there is nothing that can't be overcome through understanding and compassion.

5. During my health challenge, I want to let go of grudges, resentments, and false assumptions so I can hear the quiet guidance of my inner wisdom.

6. I am responsible for how I feel.

7. A healthy state comes as I accept myself and care for my entire being.

8. New and different situations, even ones I may call "bad" during a health challenge, are opportunities to learn.

9. What I feel is a result of my beliefs. It is important for me to take the time to see where my feelings originate.

10. Love knows no limits. We are all worthy of Love.

Exercise: The Path to Compassion, Kindness, and Gratitude

At any time we can choose to replace negative core beliefs with positive ones by turning to our inner teacher. This is actually how we direct our mind to quiet during chaos. Or we can ignore the voice within, often even unaware that we have a choice to end our suffering and discover more peace of mind. At times it may look as if you will never be free of the pain and suffering you are experiencing with your physical challenge, yet, right now, this second, you can make the decision to find peace by choosing any one of the positive core beliefs to focus on completely.

Failure to find peace while holding on to any of the negative core beliefs is inevitable. This is because you look for permanence in the impermanent, for relief where there is none, for the end of pain in the midst of fearing the future, for immortality within the fear of death. Searching for something different during a health challenge is not negative in itself. Be content and happy that you are searching, but choose wisely for what will bring you peace by reading the above lists each hour and reminding yourself that you choose between negative core beliefs and positive core beliefs. The good news is that once you set your mind toward peace and your inner teacher, and *really mean it*, everything you have sought, except for the core positive beliefs, will begin to become meaningless and hold no value or truth. Today, begin to choose to leave the insanity of the negative core beliefs and turn your mind to ideas of Truth instead. Turn to your inner teacher and ask to see a different world, awakened by your health challenge, and think a different kind of thought than those of the negative core beliefs.

For several minutes, observe your mind and see the painful world you think is real because of your health challenge. Review the thoughts and feelings which stem from these and which you think are true. Then release them, willingly, and quietly go beneath them to a place where they cannot enter. Imagine there is a door beneath all the negative core beliefs in your mind, which you can enter to discover only positive core beliefs. Know that no one can fail who seeks this door to peace. Imagine today that you have no other goal than finding this door and passing through it, and that there is nothing before this door you really want. Remember often that today is a time of gladness, and choose to refrain from negative core thoughts and endless worry. This is how to have freedom during your health challenge. Should you forget this happy fact, choose any one of the positive core beliefs and adopt it as though your freedom depends on it, because it does.

CHAPTER ELEVEN

Step Four: Practicing Wisdom Contemplation

Surrendering to Love is a particularly important practice for our entire lives. With each moment comes a new opportunity to surrender, to find the peace of the present moment, and to come to it with an empty heart, mind, and hands.

The process of asking, listening, trusting, following, and surrendering, described in this chapter, is the true purpose of intentional contemplation. If you are at all uncomfortable or awkward with the phase "intentional contemplation," feel free to replace it with the word *prayer* or *meditation*.

To be clear, this five-stage process is *not* about how to ask for what we think we want, because we are often confused about what brings us pain and what brings us joy. Instead, this process turns our lives in the direction of our inner wisdom and increases our ability to decide to follow Love's guidance during both challenging and good times. Think of this five-stage process as *wisdom contemplation.*

The Five Stages of Wisdom Contemplation

Stage One: Asking

Asking our inner wisdom for guidance is the first step of surrendering to Love in all our affairs, starting with our health challenge.

The key is to ask our inner wisdom with great intention. We should ask as if we were asking a great teacher the most important question in the world. We must want, more than anything, to hear the answer.

At times, asking with such intent—or, for that matter, even remembering to do so—may be difficult. The more we remind ourselves of the following, especially during our health challenge, the more successful we will be in finding health—peace of mind:

- I don't know the answer to this question, or what I should do in this situation.

- I believe that turning my life over to the Love within me will bring purpose, safety, meaning, success, and happiness.

- My personal judgment and ability to listen to inner wisdom can be faulty because they are wrapped in fear-based beliefs.

- Even if I don't understand the answer I hear from my inner wisdom, I will not discount it. Even if the answer scares me, I will still listen.

- I trust that my inner guidance will not result in harm to myself or others.

- All I know and all I have learned in the past may need to be set aside in order for me to follow what I hear from my inner wisdom. I am willing to do this.

- What other people think does not determine the value of my inner guidance. I am willing to go against the crowd if necessary.

❖ In following my inner guidance, I agree to do my best to release all resentment and blame.

We might resist the full impact of what will be created when we ask for inner guidance. It is important to realize that the reason we surrender to Love during a health challenge is that we have not yet found consistent peace of mind. You will find that by asking for guidance at this level, you attain the most consistent peace of mind. When we are moved to ask because we recognize the limitations of our past way of thinking and because we know our inner wisdom will answer, we take a significant stride forward on our path to health.

Stage Two: Listening

There is a significant difference between sort of listening and *truly listening with the full intention of hearing.* If you are like many people, you may have become accustomed to asking questions while already having in mind the answer that you want to hear. If you don't hear that answer, then you may either try to manipulate the answer you want into being or retreat, feeling disappointed. This type of asking and listening doesn't work very well, and it certainly does not create health.

When I was a growing up in the 1960s, a television program called *Hogan's Heroes* aired weekly. The show featured a character named Sergeant Schultz. Whenever Schultz encountered a situation requiring his input or intervention, he would loudly insist, while closing his eyes, "I know nothing. I know *nothing!*" It is helpful to say this same phrase when attempting to listen to our inner guidance. Paradoxically, recognizing that, on a judgment level, we know nothing is how we discover a deeper inner wisdom. Remember:

Often we can't hear an answer because what we think and feel about our question gets in the way.

Particularly in dealing with a health challenge, all our *shoulds* and *shouldn'ts,* concepts of right and wrong, views of health and illness, ideas, and wants and desires divert us and get in the way of us truly listening. Quieting the mind is essential if we want to be able to listen to Love.

Every word and every exercise in this book is geared toward helping us quiet ourselves and listen. As is the case with any learned skill, the more we practice quieting our mind and listening to our inner guidance, the better we become at it.

In trusting, the next stage in the process leading to surrender, we come to an important crossroads where we commit to living by Life-centered thinking rather than fear-based thinking. We can decide to listen to either the ego's harsh directives for approaching our health challenge or to the quiet, true voice of our inner wisdom.

To many, asking for inner guidance through intentional contemplation is an action not grounded in any sort of logic or reason, and taking time to ask and listen for this guidance means taking time away from finding "real" answers to our health challenge. The amazing thing is, if we were to rationally look at where our ego's fear-based judgment has led us, it would be obvious that we should not invest any of our trust in it. When we ask and listen for counsel from our inner wisdom, our overall peace of mind improves and, thus, more consistent health will flourish.

Stage Three: Trusting

A successful outcome to our health challenge can be defined as *utilizing every moment as an opportunity to learn the lessons Love is teaching us about who we are and who we are not.*

It is important to remember this definition, because too often we make the mistake of judging an outcome on the basis of what we personally think should happen, and this desired outcome is often a physical state rather than a spiritual state. This, the third stage, calls us to decide which direction we want to follow, and we make that decision based on what we place our trust in: the ego and fear-based thinking or Love and Life-centered thinking.

The choice is simple—and in wisdom contemplation during a health challenge, we say clearly to ourselves:

I choose to listen to and trust my inner wisdom. My health is not based solely on my physical state.

Stage Four: Following

When we choose Life-centered thinking, our inner guidance and outer action reflect one another. We *follow* the guidance we hear when contemplating our inner wisdom. To follow what we hear, we must trust our inner guidance. Taking any other approach will lead us to feel dragged or pushed during our health challenge, and we will usually have an edge of resentment and anger.

Though the content of our inner guidance might not seem logical or reasonable at the time, the experience that results from following it can easily stand up to reason. For example, does it not seem reasonable and logical to do whatever leads to more peace, better relationships, and the ability to be more kind?

Following is the action step of the wisdom-contemplation process. It is also the step in which we will be tempted to strike bargains. We might want to do only part of what our inner guidance says, so we try to play *Let's Make a Deal* with wisdom. The extent to which we try to bargain is the extent to which we do not trust our inner guidance.

Taking action is very simple if we trust the information we receive and very difficult if we do not. It is important that we don't allow our mind to ask too many why or what-if questions, such as "Why would I ever do that?" "What if my family doesn't agree?" "What if I lose something important to me?" or "What if I can't afford it?" *These kinds of questions are the ego's attempt to shoot holes in what we hear during wisdom contemplation.* Giving in to such questions is the reason fear often escalates during this action stage.

When we do successfully quiet ourselves and go through the steps of asking, listening, trusting, and following, a surprising thing happens: Our inner guidance does not always prompt us to do anything different. Instead, it leads us to work with our thoughts in ways that create more peace. At first working on our thoughts during a physical health challenge can seem crazy, because for so many people, health is limited to the body. And even when we trust our inner wisdom, our health challenges may not change in the ways we want. Yet, our inner wisdom can bring us answers about who we really are, and with this comes peace, clarity, and purpose.

Stage Five: Surrendering

Although following what we hear from our inner wisdom is important, it is still shy of complete surrender. Though any aspects of saying yes to Life can be difficult during our health challenge, practicing surrender can be particularly trying.

The good news is that surrender is within us, wanting to move through us like a gently flowing river. Most of us experienced a type of surrender as children. I remember carrying my kids when they were a year or two old. They cuddled close to me in total trust. They would sleep in my arms, surrendering in the moment, knowing without a doubt that they were being held in safety and in love. When during a health challenge I have successfully surrendered to Love in the same way, I have had my fullest experiences of true peace, even in the midst of physical illness and pain.

Practicing directing our minds toward Love on a daily basis is of paramount importance, no matter how we are feeling physically or what our symptoms are. This is how the mind is quieted. If we are speeding through one task or treatment after the other during our health challenge, we tend to go on autopilot. And when we slip into this mode, we are trying to have the world go according to our plan. We are at war with what is.

Surrender can be described as accepting what is and accepting it from a place of Love—being completely present with the way things are in the moment *and* inviting Love into the moment. The times that I have been able to surrender completely have been the result of seeing that worry, suffering, and unhappiness come from not wanting things to be the way they are—not wanting my body to be as it is, not wanting people in my life to be how they are, not wanting myself to be how I am, not wanting my situation to be how it is, not wanting the world to be as it is.

Certain thoughts and beliefs keep us from surrendering. Not unlike many others, I had struggled much of my life with the uncomfortable and damaging emotions of anger, jealousy, pettiness, envy, and so on. Surrender cannot coexist with these emotions. Over the course of thirty years, I have undertaken many therapeutic approaches, practiced different meditations, gone to workshops, and read books. After all these efforts, I can tell you that what is the highest truth can be said in one simple sentence:

> *When I become angry, jealous, petty, envious, and so forth, it is always because I am wanting some person, some thing, some body, or some situation to be different than it is in that moment, and peace of mind eludes me.*

Surrender is about learning to be present with what is *while resting in the grace of Love.* This is the purest of health goals and the most profound path to Love. Surrender leads to a much simpler life than one in which we're slaves of the ego's constant cravings, desires, and striving. It also brings a unique peace during our most challenging health challenges.

When it comes to surrendering, I am far from perfect. But if, when I find myself upset, I pause, breathe, and focus on accepting the way things are (or, more to the point, stop wanting things to be different) *and* on feeling the presence of Love, I experience peace. In contrast, when I get worked up about the way things are, don't turn to Love, and constantly try by my sheer will or blind hope to make things different,

I am heading for guaranteed conflict, increased stress, and decreased health.

It may sound as if surrendering means never wanting to accomplish anything, to improve our physical health, or to work at making the world a better place. Nothing could be further from the truth.

Surrender allows us to come to the moment, unencumbered by our past and fear-based thinking, in order to experience the only want that has any meaning: *wanting the peace of Love.* In this way, surrender brings us back to what is most real. Experiencing even moments of surrender to Love, we discover what it is like to *really* want something important and valuable. The paradox is that when we stop wanting our situation to be different from a place of fear and attachment, and instead have the single goal of wanting the peace that Love bestows, then we are able to actually make a profound difference. Thus, the steps discussed in this book can be seen as circular, but always advancing in depth.

Summary of the Five Stages of Wisdom Contemplation

Here is a summary of each of the five stages of wisdom contemplation. In italics are statements you can make in order to put wisdom contemplation into action, beginning right now. I suggest writing down this summary or keeping it handy, and undertaking wisdom contemplation on a daily basis. It is always good to start your day with it, and if possible, to do it several times throughout your day.

1. **Ask** your inner wisdom for direction in your life and protection from your own fear-based thinking during your

health challenge. *My way is fearful and won't work well. I humbly ask for new direction and care in my life.*

2. **Listen** with the full intent to hear your inner wisdom and with a willingness to let go of your preconceived ideas about health, outcomes, and what you think you want. *In order to listen in each moment to my inner wisdom rather than to fear, I am willing to let go of what I have thought I wanted and needed.*

3. **Trust** that this time in your life is an opportunity to learn the lessons Love is teaching. *I trust that each and every day during my health challenge has a lesson for me—an opportunity to learn more of love and compassion and of how to extend understanding and empathy.*

4. **Follow** the guidance of your inner wisdom, being certain that it will bring you peace and healing. Have the courage to take action in your life when guided to do so and to be still when guided to do so. *I commit to putting Love's guidance into action in my life. These actions are, in the most literal sense, labors of Love. Stillness can be an action as well.*

5. **Surrender** by being present with what is while resting in the grace of Love. *I surrender to the present moment, and I find and share Love's tenderness.*

CHAPTER TWELVE

Step Five: Getting Better

The period following the most difficult part of a health challenge can be very frustrating unless we recognize it as another stage of saying yes to Life. This time can be problematic because we begin to realize that though we might be getting better physically, the road ahead is not going to be short or easy, and our ongoing condition or the aftereffects of our health challenge may affect many parts of our life for the long term.

Wanting to experience a good life following a health challenge is a worthy goal. The problem is that most people are very confused about what a good life might look like. For those who regain their previous physical health, forgetting the health challenge ever happened and going on with life may seem like a good idea. For those who haven't regained their previous physical health, stress and loss can plague their lives. The key factor to both is that those who truly have posttraumatic growth are those who consciously continue to deepen their learning no matter what.

Saying yes to Life doesn't end when our health challenge does. Rather, getting better is the next stage in our posttraumatic growth.

Understanding Power

To fully understand the "getting better" stage of saying yes to Life, we must first understand what power is and is not.

Fear-based thinking associates three words with the idea of power: *control, dominate,* and *accumulate.* The ego tells us that power is what makes and keeps us safe and happy. It defines power as the ability to control our environment, our body, and all situations; to dominate whenever possible; and to accumulate as much material wealth as possible. But contrary to what many people believe, this is *not* power. *True power is being aware of who we are, being in touch with our inner wisdom, being present in the moment, and being Life-centered.*

Posttraumatic growth lies in seeing the connectedness of all life, not in controlling all life. As many of the martial arts teach, power is often found in yielding rather than dominating, and our ability to respond powerfully to a situation is deterred by any thinking that takes us away from being completely in the moment. We experience true power and healing when we choose to see the truth about who we are, no matter what our physical condition or the trauma we may have recently experienced. We are powerful when we have the intention to heal rather than to remain in fear; healing comes from the direction of our inner wisdom, while fear comes from our perceived helplessness. Life-centered thinking leads us to understand true power and experience posttraumatic growth.

The following table outlines these two distinctly different approaches to power and healing and to the development of posttraumatic growth.

Views of Healing and Power

Fear-Based Thinking *(Limits Posttraumatic Growth)*	Life-Centered Thinking *(Develops Posttraumatic Growth)*
1. Control at all cost.	1. Release the past.
2. The end result is more important than the inner process.	2. Giving and receiving in the present moment are the basis of health and healing.
3. Analyze every situation.	3. Accept that which you cannot change.
4. Judge your body.	4. See beyond your body.
5. Never admit a mistake.	5. Embrace your humanness.
6. Dominate all.	6. Accept what is and know there is a lesson from Love in what is.
7. Accumulate as much as possible.	7. Share as much as possible.
8. If you think you are being threatened, attack, fight, and win.	8. Forgive.
9. Figure out the future.	9. Be present in the moment.
10. Always have a good defense.	10. Trust in your inner wisdom and practice surrendering to Love.

Moving Beyond Limitations

Do you want your health challenge to make you better or bitter? In asking yourself this question, you are asking whether you want to live in a world of limitation or a world of possibility and opportunities to give and receive love.

As you look at any limitations of your body after a health challenge and conclude that because of them, your life will not be a happy one, ask yourself:

◆ Is this conclusion what Love wants me to have?

◆ Is this conclusion the truth about who I am?

◆ Do I want this limiting belief?

◆ What does this belief do to my awareness of the power of Love within me?

In honestly answering these questions, you are taking the step necessary to allow yourself to move beyond limitation and enter posttraumatic growth, even as you move beyond the worst of your health challenge.

Each day, part of my path is choosing to see a world where I am no longer limited in happiness or helpless in any way and one where I have no enemies—only people and situations that teach me more about letting go of any upset and finding empathy and understanding. As I make this choice, the means of healing become available to me. Though I am not yet always able to perfectly view the world this way, simply having the intention to do so makes my life so much better than when I blindly give in to fear-based thinking.

Following the most difficult parts of a health challenge, deciding to continue to look within and to surrender to Love brings a sense of relief and a feeling of calm. Recognizing the truth of who we are in Love's eyes adds a dimension of consistency to a life that may have been chaotic.

Deciding What You Are

If we truly want to hear the still, quiet voice within, it will not be drowned out by all the concerns or pain we experience during our health challenge. However, our ability to fully find posttraumatic growth depends on our belief in what we are.

If, after the most difficult parts of a physical health challenge, we choose to go back to listening to and following what fear tells us, we will ultimately see ourselves as fragile, afraid, and vulnerable. As a result, we'll experience depression, low self-esteem, a chronic feeling of worthlessness, and often intense loneliness. We will believe we are helpless. Even though we may look like we are very much in control, or we may put on a smile for the world, we will believe that our mind and our body are weak. We will believe that the condition of our body dictates how we should feel and react and that outside forces determine how we feel.

But there is an alternative.

The Alternative to Suffering and Limitation

There is a way
of being in the world
that is beyond all your problems
and beyond all concerns
of your body.
Choose to listen
to another voice.

The voice of Love and kindness whispers
that you are one with all that is.
Surrender to this voice
and your goal to have true health,
peace of mind,
is accomplished.

By listening to the guidance of Love, we remind ourselves that we are safe and that the power of Love can truly heal our minds. We extend compassion rather than building defenses or perpetuating worry. Our self-esteem is high because we see no value in beating ourselves up, identifying ourselves with our body, or holding on to shame. We feel worthwhile because we recognize the value in each and every living being. We do not feel helpless or out of control, because we recognize that our thinking and our values are totally ours to choose. Our thoughts, not the situation, determine our experience. We recognize that there is nothing in the universe any more powerful than our thinking when we surrender to Love.

As we move beyond the storm of emotions and treatments that accompany health challenges, the difference in the questions asked by fear-based thinking and Life-centered thinking points to a fundamental difference in beliefs. Fear-based questions assume that Love exists in some places and not in others; that it exists for some people, but not for others; that it exists in some times, but not in other times. There is a belief that we must *do* something in order to *get* better rather than seeing the Love that is within us right now. This set of false assumptions makes it very difficult to surrender to Love, which is the basis for posttraumatic growth, for at best we believe surrendering would be a hit-or-miss experience.

In contrast, Life-centered thinking directs us to look within for what might be blocking our awareness of Love, and it sets us on the course for posttraumatic growth. Life-centered thinking assumes and believes that Love exists at all times and in all places. It is only our mind that can create obstacles to our ability to experience Love, and our mind is independent of the condition of our body.

Regardless of what we may have believed, *everything we struggled with during our health challenge—including depression, failure, and feelings of being stuck in misery—came from the belief that we are separate from Love and that we don't have the choice or opportunity to experience peace.*

There is certainly no single way that we adopt this health-inhibiting belief and the feelings of powerlessness that come as a result. However, there is one way to rise above them.

Those who find their way out of helplessness and misery and into posttraumatic growth ask themselves some very powerful and important questions. In answering these questions, they are redefining who they are, which is a key motivator for posttraumatic growth. If we believe we are alone and separated from Love in a cruel and harsh world, we will not be motivated to surrender to Love's guidance; at best, we will be motivated to try to control our surroundings and our body in order to minimize our pain.

Each of the questions below has a large subset of questions, and each requires some deep inner searching to answer. The full exploration of these questions can take quite some time, because posttraumatic growth is an ongoing process—not something we do once and are done with, not something that ends when our health challenge ends. It can be beneficial to have a friend, therapist, minister, or coach or mentor help you address these questions.

Of the many life-changing questions that form the basis for posttraumatic growth, here are the four primary ones:

◈ Do I desire a life that I rule by choosing to surrender to Love, instead of one where the world and the condition of my body rule me?

◈ Do I desire a life in which I am powerful because I identify myself with Love rather than helpless because I identify myself as only a body?

◈ Do I desire a life in which I have no enemies or dreaded situations, only teachers to show how to increase understanding and empathy?

◈ Do I want to see all the beauty I have denied myself or overlooked, and see the truth of who I am?

We cannot be powerful, heal, or become "better" and at the same time be afraid of who we are. Those who attempt this combination usually become one or more of what I term the four *D*s: depressed, dominating, dogmatic, and dictatorial.

When we try to be powerful and maintain our health while fearing who we are, because we believe we are someone other than whom Love created us to be, we will always try to control or conquer our outside world, and we will always overidentify with the condition of our body. For some, after the most difficult parts of a health challenge, this fear is turned outward, and they become dogmatic and dominating, often growing increasingly difficult to live with because they become dictatorial. For others, the fear is turned inward, causing them to cower from their own potential, feel helpless, and limit themselves in every way, eventually becoming depressed.

Do not let irrational fears and the four Ds keep you from asking and fully answering the important questions above, for these questions are key to posttraumatic growth.

The Power of Willingness

To practice turning to our inner wisdom and Love in all our healing, we need to continue developing a willingness to do so, especially during difficult times. Willingness is a subtle but powerful tool of the mind and can be used to begin to uproot the ego. Think for a moment of somebody who is furiously arguing a point but is clearly mistaken and does not have the full picture of the truth. They are very entrenched in being right about what they believe and cannot listen or see reality because they are so locked into one way of seeing the situation. Think of the possible shift that could occur, the doors that could open, if this person were to pause in a calm manner, take a couple of minutes, and say the simple words, "I may be mistaken. I am willing to see this situation differently."

Similarly, during a health challenge our inner teacher can offer a perspective leading to posttraumatic growth, but only if we are willing to have such a shift in our perception, only if we hold in our mind the powerful tool of "I am willing to see this situation differently than through fear and worry."

The best way to begin cultivating that willingness is to realize how our healing and happiness have been inhibited because of the compulsion to analyze and judge. When we see negative judgments, comparisons, and fear as what they are, roadblocks to inner peace, *we will be more willing* to let them go and turn to Love.

Exercise: Develop the
Power of Willingness

Asking our inner wisdom for guidance and being willing to surrender to its guidance are a *process* rather than an *act,* because they encompass several steps. Eventually this process becomes more automatic and is incorporated into our daily lives, but at first, we must become willing to have a perspective different from the one the fearful ego offers us. The power of willingness, which is a persistent force in overcoming the ego, can begin this moment to help you say yes to Life.

Spend a few minutes each hour today observing your mind for all its judgments and negative thoughts about your health challenge, and then say, "I may be mistaken. I am now willing to see this all differently." Then turn your attention to your inner teacher and listen. Simply listen. Say a few times to yourself, "I am willing to listen to my inner teacher." This may seem repetitive or awkward, but it is truly a spiritual practice in undoing the ego and its view of your health challenge. The words "I am willing to see this differently," are the beginning of any deeply meaningful life.

CHAPTER THIRTEEN

Step Six: Deepening Wisdom Contemplation

Practicing wisdom contemplation is a part of steps four and six of saying yes to Life because even as our physical health challenge resolves, it remains the foundation of our continued healing and posttraumatic growth. The deepening of a practice of wisdom contemplation first helps us gain a different perspective of our health challenge and later becomes the foundation for an ongoing development of living a purposeful life.

To help you continue using the five stages of wisdom contemplation (described in chapter eleven), we will now explore four phases for developing your wisdom contemplation. These four phases embody many of the details already discussed, but this time, I will show you how to employ wisdom contemplation for continued, post–health challenge healing.

Four Phases of Developing Wisdom Contemplation

Phase One: Acknowledging That There Is Another Way

Our ego hates the phrase "There is another way," because when we utter it, we are saying we believe that there is a power greater than fear, even greater than technology, that has far more wisdom than our ego. Most of us like to think that our way is the right way, and we can be pretty darn resistant to saying there must be a better way. Regardless of our resistance, the time has come to make the declaration, because it is the foundation of wisdom contemplation and for posttraumatic growth.

Wisdom contemplation directs our mind toward posttraumatic growth by seeing the "something better" beyond the condition of our bodies. Practicing wisdom contemplation every day is essentially holding up a stop sign in front of our fear-based thinking. By practicing wisdom contemplation, we firmly tell our mind, "I am not going to trust my ego and fear-based thinking any further when it comes to health." To initiate wisdom contemplation, we must at least be willing to say "There must be a better and more peaceful way of going through my health challenge and through my life than always listening to my fear-based thinking."

Many of us have to experience a type of hitting bottom, before we surrender to our inner wisdom. Hitting bottom is when we finally see that the way of fear-based thinking has not served us, and it sometimes comes when we receive difficult news about a physical condition. Even after we have begun to accept what is happening, there is usually a time when we again feel very unsettled. This time is the opportunity to turn anew to our inner wisdom, which leads to more surrender.

At this point, inner conflict can be great. We ask ourselves, "How can I have done so much to heal and get healthy, yet still be in such pain and still be unhappy?" Despair increases, and for a while, hope decreases. Then, if we choose, we can finally become truly willing to see that there is another way to view our health challenge.

Typically, this turbulent stage is not a onetime occurrence. I remember dropping into this despair years after I became deaf. Knowing there is a better way allowed me to begin reflecting on my situation again. Was I continuing to turn to Love? Was I again attempting to handle things without a spiritual focus? Was I continuing to forgive? Was I inspiring anybody by demonstrating Life-centered living?

As you go to sleep each night, no matter where you are in the process of dealing with your health challenge, make the commitment that tomorrow you will make saying yes to Life your most important goal. As you drift to sleep, say this one short sentence:

I will wake up knowing there is a better way, a way to feel and demonstrate Love.

Phase Two: Turning Away from the Ego by Quieting Your Mind

When we acknowledge that there must be a better way to live, our ego will still loudly proclaim that we are crazy to turn away from its guidance. To move on in our healing, we need to not only be willing to turn away from fear-based thinking, but also practice quieting our mind and ignoring the chatter of the ego. Sometimes this practice can feel as if we are running against a strong wind, because progress can be slow and laborious, especially when all has been turned upside down in our world. We must be willing to persevere despite any perceived setbacks. The ego's voice often dominates when the chips are down, and it can take some time to be able to consistently quiet our mind.

The core of wisdom contemplation is the ability to quiet the mind and listen to our inner wisdom with complete awareness in the present moment. Like any task, this one takes dedication and persistence to master.

The following exercises present techniques you can use to begin the practice of quieting your mind on a daily basis, thus setting the stage for peace of mind. Try them all and then choose one or two that work best for you. Continue with those awhile before switching to other techniques.

At first glance, some of these methods may seem awkward or silly. If they do, remember that you have had a great deal of education in analytical thought but probably not many lessons on how to stop habitual negative thinking and silence the ego's chatter. Though the act of quieting your mind may seem foreign, it's a necessary step in continued healing, because it allows you listen to your inner wisdom without distraction.

For all the techniques, you may start out with five-minute practice periods, but then it is helpful to work up to about twenty minutes. Remember, the key is practice. The more you focus on quieting your mind, the more you will find a peaceful feeling resulting from it. Try not to give in to any initial frustration.

Exercise: Quieting the Mind with Conscious Breathing

The breath is a powerful tool for quieting the mind, especially when there is physical discomfort. Sit or lie comfortably with your back erect yet relaxed. Lay your hands loosely by your sides or fold them in your lap.

With your eyes closed, begin by simply observing your breath. Do not try to change your breathing in any way; simply watch it.

After a few minutes, check to see if your breath is full and extending into your abdomen. If not, deepen your breathing. Each cycle of breath should be slow, smooth, and uninterrupted.

As you watch your breath, you may notice that it is difficult to keep your mind from racing from thought to thought or to keep focused on your body. Simply bring your focus back to your breathing whenever you find yourself stuck on an unwanted thought. Imagine that with each exhalation, you can release more of your thoughts.

Focus on one aspect of your breath. For example, place your attention on the pause between when you inhale and exhale—the time when you are not quite inhaling but not yet exhaling either. Do not stop your breathing; just focus your attention on this pause. Or you can focus your attention on the soft, barely audible sound your breathing makes. Another point of focus might be the area between your upper lip and nose, where you can feel the air entering and exiting your nostrils.

Exercise: Quieting the Mind with a Word or Statement

Focusing on one statement, repeated over and over, lets all other thoughts slip away. By placing your focus on one particular word or idea, you enable yourself to move *inward* with it.

Though the specific word or phrase you choose can vary, it is important to use one that does not carry negative messages. To begin with, I suggest that on your inhale, you use, "I am," and on your exhale use, "relaxed."

Alternatively, many people have found repeating the word *one* to be helpful for focusing their attention.

With your eyes closed and your breathing relaxed and deep, begin to silently repeat to yourself the phrase or word you have chosen. You can attach the word or phrase to each inhalation and exhalation. For example, if using the word *one*, say "One," as you inhale and then again as you exhale.

If you find yourself sidetracked or thinking about something else, gently bring your attention back to your word or statement.

Exercise: Quieting the Mind with Walking Meditation

Because walking is often a part of the physical recovery from a health challenge, many people find a walking meditation helpful. This technique allows you to move yet is very quieting and centering as well. Walking meditation has been an enormous benefit to my healing and spiritual practice.

Walking meditation is about slowing down and finding the stillness in you and the joy that lives in that stillness. Start out by walking slowly, with a pace that feels relaxed. As you walk, exhale long and slow. The breath will be drawn naturally back into your body. As thoughts arise, turn your attention back to the full exhale.

Walking through a quiet neighborhood or park is preferred over walking along a busy street. Walking in this manner for fifteen to thirty minutes daily will bring wonderful benefits that will enrich your life.

Some simple variations worth exploring: Walk with your hands clasped together, as in seated meditation. Walk with awareness of each foot as it touches the earth. Walk with your head slightly bowed. As you walk, imagine leaving a flower on the ground beneath each step. Walk as if you were an enlightened being fully in the present moment, with no random thoughts about anything else. Walk with a gentle smile on your lips. Walk to a rhythm created by counting steps on your inhale and exhale.

Exercise: Quieting the Mind with Thought Naming

This approach is particularly helpful for those who say "No matter what I do, I just can't control my thoughts, I am too preoccupied with my health challenge." The previous three approaches are used to focus your attention. This thought-naming approach is based on the same principle, but here you use the thoughts themselves to focus your attention.

With this technique, instead of fighting and controlling your thoughts, you simply watch and name them as they come and go. As you do, it is important to maintain a detached mental stance. Simply observe your thoughts and tell yourself what each thought is about. Watch your thoughts as if you were watching a movie, with the task of naming each scene and then going on to the next.

Let's imagine, for example, that you are sitting with your eyes closed, and you begin to think about test results that are coming. Say to yourself, "Thinking about the test results," and then go on to whatever else pops into your mind. Try not to delve into any one thought. Just name it and go on to the next. The practice of remaining detached from each thought will allow you to become mentally still.

Exercise: Quieting the Mind with an External Focus

We have all experienced staring into a fire and becoming mesmerized by the flickering flames. In this approach, you use an external object to focus your attention. Once your thoughts are quiet, you can continue to turn within. Though any object will do, even a spot on the wall or a star in the sky, the single flame of a candle is an easy object to practice with because it is so captivating.

When looking at the flame, allow yourself to focus all of your attention on it, as if it were the only thing in the entire world. Don't take your eyes off of it. You may find it helpful to repeat the phrase "My mind is still" or "Watching the flame" as you concentrate on the candle.

Exercise: Quieting the Mind with Physical Focusing

With this approach, the body is the object of your attention. Through a combination of the walking meditation and thought-naming exercise, you focus on any body sensation, even pain or a symptom you don't like, while avoiding becoming attached to it. This technique it is also an excellent tool for controlling pain.

It is only when you become future oriented that the discomfort begins to control you. When you begin to think, "When is this pain going to stop?" or "I can't take this anymore" (be it physical or emotional pain), you become captive to the discomfort. Conversely, when you acknowledge the discomfort or pain in the present moment without extending it into the future, it ceases to have power over you.

If you have ever experienced a sudden onset of pain, such as hitting your finger with a hammer, you know that your mind is not thinking about a lot of things in that moment other than the pain. In this approach, you use a lesser degree of discomfort—or for that matter, a pleasurable sensation—to your advantage and use body sensations as a means of focusing your attention and quieting your mind.

Phase Three: Practicing Nonattachment

It's important to understand what guidance from our inner wisdom is and what it is not. In chapter eleven's discussion on *asking,* the first stage of wisdom contemplation, a series of questions was presented to help you ask for guidance in a genuine and deep way. Let's expand on this idea by exploring the concept of nonattachment—the willingness to come to Love with empty hands and an open heart, at all stages of our healing.

Our culture tends to be very results oriented, especially when it comes to the body. From standardized testing in schools to bathroom scales at home to medical approaches for dealing with a disease, we are constantly looking for tangible and external indicators of progress. Although this kind of measurement can offer useful information, far too much emphasis can be placed on external measurement. *The overvaluing of outside measurements is a key factor in unhappiness and stress, especially during a health challenge.*

Life-centered thinking does not view time in the same way fear-based thinking does. Therefore, when we ask for guidance from our inner wisdom and move toward surrender, we may hear a direction that has no apparent measurable value. Here we must trust that listening to our inner wisdom will result in a positive outcome. Remember, the primary goal of wisdom contemplation is always peace of mind, and this peace can always come when we surrender to Love.

Furthermore, our ego tends to ask questions with the answer it wants to hear already in mind. It "contemplates" this way as well. Nonattachment—the willingness to come to Love without thinking we know what should happen—is a central focus of wisdom contemplation.

In scientific research, there is a phenomenon known as experimenter bias, in which the experimenter's beliefs influence what he or she will find. Even in the most controlled situations, the preconceived ideas of what the results will be can influence the outcome. In the same way, when we ask for guidance, we must identify and attempt to set aside any preconceived ideas.

The most significant discoveries I have made in my life have come from turning to Love during a health challenge with empty hands, a quiet mind, and an open heart. When I have supported myself in this process, I have always found purpose and meaning where only confusion, suffering, and fear existed previously.

Phase Four: Directing Your Mind to Listen, Trust, and Surrender

In chapter eleven, we have already discussed listening, trusting, and surrendering. The following are guidelines to ensure that you are able to listen to your inner wisdom during all phases of dealing with a health challenge. They serve as a basis for your continued healing journey and will help you trust what you hear from your inner wisdom. I suggest you read these guidelines before you enter periods of contemplation. If over time some guidelines seem particularly helpful, use them to start your wisdom-contemplation sessions each day.

Guidelines for Trusting and Following Wisdom Contemplation

1. Refrain from judging what you see on the surface.

2. Do not ask a question and then plug your ears because you're afraid of the answer.

3. Remember that you do not have to understand something in order for it to have truth.

4. With your inner wisdom, don't listen and judge. Instead, listen and trust.

5. You naturally hear your inner wisdom as you let go of fear.

6. You cannot listen to Love while condemning yourself.

7. You cannot blame others and listen to Love.

8. See possibilities for healing instead of obstacles to Love and forgiveness.

9. Set aside other people's voices so you can hear your inner wisdom.

10. Listen with empty hands, a quiet mind, and an open heart.

11. Trust in what creates connection, not in what creates separation.

12. Remember that you cannot really listen to your inner wisdom as long as you hold on to expectations or specific outcomes to situations.

13. Keep in mind that you cannot be impatient and be able to really listen. Trust Love's timing more than your timing.

14. It is most difficult to trust and surrender while holding on to the past.

15. Only when you're willing to let go of old beliefs can you fully listen.

16. To be able to listen, trust, and surrender, you cannot remain attached to being right.

17. Assumptions about yourself and others cloud your ability to hear.

18. If you believe you are alone in a world of scarcity, you will generally look for information to support this belief, and surrender to Love will be difficult.

19. It is hard to listen, trust, and surrender if you focus on the condition of your body or what you are going to get from your inner wisdom.

20. It is impossible to listen and trust when you have a closed mind. You must believe that anything is possible and that there are no limitations on yourself or others.

21. Guidance always includes forgiveness. If you place value in attack and defense, you will not be able to trust your guidance or surrender fully to it.

22. If you see yourself as weak, you will think that your guidance is asking more of you than you can give, and you will not trust it.

In Closing

After covering a large amount of ground, let us end with simplicity.

During a health challenge, we can become overwhelmed with the tasks at hand and the suffering that may accompany our journey. Remember that during these times it is important to work on our own inner peace, our healing, in addition to any medical treatment.

The real key to consistent peace of mind is finding the incredibly good things in the seemingly small things, each moment, every day: the way the sun hits a flower, the kindness of someone who did not know we were watching, the feeling in our heart when we extend love or give in some way. We can notice these things no matter how our health challenge progresses, if we choose.

This is not to discount that in our humanness, even when we are saying yes to Life, we can become sad and overwhelmed, or we may want to enjoy a bit of splendor in good news. But it is important not to let ourselves be taken from the small miracles of each day. They are there for us, and they begin in our own perception. They are the source of all healing.

At some point in life, most of us will face health challenges of some kind. Now may be your time, or it may be in the future. Some would call this view a negative or fatalistic attitude. I call it a realistic view of existence with a body. And since we all come into this world with a body, we all might as well be prepared to learn and grow from a health challenge when it comes.

Many of the ideas I have shared with you I encountered throughout my three decades of studying and practicing psychology, my own serious spiritual path, and my own personal growth through surviving and then thriving after severe and recurrent health challenges. I have studied many of the world's spiritual traditions, contemporary psychologies, and medical research on the effects of stress, negative emotion, and lack of forgiveness on our health. I did so in the hope of finding answers for myself, guidance I could share with the people with whom I work, and, ultimately, information to bring to a wider audience via the book you hold in your hands.

But as I write this today, the truth is that none of this information matters to me in the way it used to. All that matters is that you, the person reading this sentence right now, feel understood and encouraged. As I imagine you reading this book, I also imagine all the various scenarios and challenges you may be facing, and I extend love, compassion, and kindness to you across time and space, to whenever and wherever you are reading. I believe this outreach makes a difference, however subtle, for both of us.

Lastly, I reach out from my heart to the place within you that knows, to some degree, that you can grow from any challenge. This knowledge is more valuable than any information that your mind can accumulate.

In this spirit, I close with a poem I wrote as I contemplated one of my most challenging times.

Freedom Beyond Fear

I was tired
of being sick,
afraid,
and uncertain.

Would I look back
over the varied terrain of my life
and see it had all been pointless?

I am glad I asked.
It made me look for new answers
—to the very place I thought was my enemy.

I became the student,
my illness the teacher,
rather than the villain it was a moment before.

If my life is to be of use,
to have meaning,
this day and each that follows,
however many or few,
I will live as though today were the last
and held the answers to all eternity.
I will love
even when worry and fear
scream penetratingly.
I will look deeply into what is happening
rather than only wishing for something that is not
happening.

I find what is forever free and beautiful
waiting patiently within
even during this challenge.

List of Exercises

List of Key Concepts

About the Author

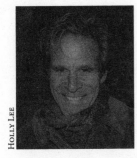

HOLLY LEE

LEE JAMPOLSKY is a recognized leader in the field of psychology and human potential. He is best known for his work on creating positive attitude, decreasing stress, setting and obtaining goals, motivating individuals and teams, and achieving peak performance. He is the author of several previous books, including *Smile for No Good Reason, Healing the Addictive Personality,* and *Healing the Addictive Mind.*

Dr. Jampolsky, or Dr. Lee as he is increasingly known, has served on the medical staff and faculty of respected hospitals and graduate schools, helped individuals around the globe, and consulted with management and CEOs of businesses of all sizes. He has appeared on numerous radio and television shows around the globe and has been interviewed or quoted in the *Wall Street Journal, BusinessWeek,* the *Los Angeles Times, Woman's World,* and other notable publications.

Dr. Lee welcomes your interest in his work. For the latest, please visit his website at *www.DrLeeJampolsky.com.*